THE
MEDITERRANEAN
ZONE

Unleash the Power of the World's Healthiest Diet for Superior Weight Loss, Health, and Longevity

THE
Mediterranean
ZONE

BARRY SEARS, PH.D.

Z
ZINC
INK

BALLANTINE BOOKS

NEW YORK

No book can replace the diagnostic expertise and medical advice of a trusted physician. Please be certain to consult with your doctor before making any decisions that affect your health or extreme changes in your diet, particularly if you suffer from any medical condition or have any symptom that may require treatment.

Published in the United States by Zinc Ink, an imprint of Random House, a division of Random House LLC, a Penguin Random House Company, New York.

BALLANTINE and the HOUSE colophon are registered trademarks of Random House LLC.
ZINC INK is a trademark of David Zinczenko.

LIBRARY OF CONGRESS CATALOGING-IN-PUBLICATION DATA
Sears, Barry.
The Mediterranean zone : unleash the power of the world's healthiest diet for superior weight loss, health, and longevity / Barry Sears , Ph.D.
pages   cm
Includes bibliographical references and index.
ISBN 978-0-8041-7917-1
eBook ISBN 978-0-8041-7919-5
1. Reducing diets. 2. Diet—Mediterranean Region. 3. Diet therapy—Mediterranean Region. 4. Inflammation—Diet therapy. 5. Weight loss. 6. Longevity. 7. Nutrition. 8. Health. I. Title.
RM222.2.S3893 2014
613.2′5—dc23   2014026641

Printed in the United States of America on acid-free paper

www.ballantinebooks.com

2 4 6 8 9 7 5 3 1

First Edition

Book design by Caroline Cunningham

To Hippocrates, who was right when he said,

"Let food be your medicine, and let medicine be your food."

Contents

Preface

The United Nations has declared the Mediterranean diet a historical treasure. The Mayo Clinic recommends it as a way to combat heart disease and Alzheimer's. The *New England Journal of Medicine* has reported time and again on the medical benefits of the Mediterranean diet. Health and beauty magazines constantly tout the Mediterranean diet's effectiveness.

Yet, somehow, no one can really describe it. How many calories a day do you need to maintain your weight on the Mediterranean diet? No one knows. How much protein per day do you need to be on the Mediterranean diet? No one knows. What is the right balance of protein to carbohydrate on the Mediterranean diet? No one knows. Why does it really work? No one knows.

This fuzzy thinking is what passes for nutritional knowledge in America today. A lot of talk, a lot of hype, but with very little true understanding behind those words. Nutrition is complex, but complex doesn't attract page views or sell magazines. What actually gains public attention are simple solutions (especially concerning the elimination of "evil" foods) easily put into sound bytes that resonate on TV but have little scientific basis.

But the Mediterranean diet can't be reduced to simple rules such as "don't eat red meat" or "drink red wine." And for that reason, many people believe that having a glass of wine with their pasta means they're following the Mediterranean diet.

If you can unlock the true nature of the Mediterranean diet—if you can identify the factors that make it work—you can begin to make an enormous impact on your health starting today. And if you understand how this traditional diet works, you can refine it and take it to a much higher level to generate even greater health benefits, including the most elusive of them all for most Americans: permanent weight control.

The Mediterranean Zone represents the evolution of the Mediterranean diet into a cohesive dietary program that provides not only the structure needed for maximum health benefits, but also offers the simple rules that make it easy to use in your daily life. The Mediterranean Zone also represents a return to the past to bring the accumulated folklore of the Mediterranean diet into the twenty-first century. In many ways, the preface of *The Mediterranean Zone* could have easily been written by Hippocrates 2,500 years ago when he said, "Let food be your medicine, and let medicine be your food." Yet to truly understand his wisdom requires an understanding of the recent advances in molecular biology (gene transcription factors, epigenetics, and so on) that explain why the Mediterranean diet has such a powerful impact on one's health.

Although the science behind the Mediterranean Zone is robust, most people only care about (1) what's it in for them and (2) how easily it can be incorporated into their hassled life. So let's go right to the bottom line: What's in it for you is an extraordinary litany of life-altering benefits, including freedom from heart disease, diabetes, and other modern scourges; a dramatic reduction in your risk of Alzheimer's and other diseases of aging; younger, healthier-looking skin; and permanent weight control. And as far as its ease of use, this book breaks it all down into a plan that's so simple, all you need is one hand, one eye, and a watch. If you have those three things, you can reap the benefits of the Mediterranean Zone for a lifetime.

Introduction

The Zone at 20

When I wrote my first book, *The Zone*, in 1995, I was careful not to use the word *diet* in the title. In fact, the book was written for cardiologists to alert them to the power of food to alter hormonal responses, especially those hormones involved in inflammation. The book was meant as a clarion call to the medical community that the low-fat, high-carbohydrate diet being recommended to the American public by the medical establishment was going to lead to epidemics of obesity and diabetes driven by increased inflammation. Not inflammation caused by a microbe or an injury, but inflammation caused by what we were eating.

The focus of *The Zone* was on a little known group of hormones called eicosanoids. Even though the 1982 Nobel Prize in Medicine was awarded for understanding the importance of these hormones in driving inflammation, outside of a few in academic medicine, by 1995 still virtually no one knew anything about them.

I knew that getting attention for the book was going to be a challenge, and my publisher readily agreed. So neither of us was surprised that the initial sales of *The Zone* were modest and quickly petered out. I was convinced that the right message wasn't getting across, and that the media were looking at this book as just another fad diet book. Recklessly (without telling my wife), I went in search of a publicity firm that could help reposition the message of *The Zone*.

Since I grew up in Los Angeles, I figured if you could publicize films, you probably could do the same for books—even technical books on diet-induced inflammation. (Talk about being naïve.) So I went to the top PR firm in Hollywood and asked them if they had ever publicized a book. Their answer was no, but they were not willing turn a client away, so Michael Keaton's press agent became the head of their new book publicity department with me as their first client.

I told them the only way I could judge their efforts was by any increase in book sales (which wouldn't be too hard). Not much happened at first, but with only about four more weeks to go before my money ran out, I caught a break when Dennis Prager, a prominent LA radio talk show host, agreed to have me on his program because we both shared the same publisher. Although he liked the book, he made it clear that if there weren't any callers in the first fifteen minutes, he would have to take me off the air. I told him I was just happy to get a chance to discuss the book. Three hours later, the phone lines were still jammed with callers, and I was still on the show. The book became the #1 best seller in Los Angeles the next week and a month later the #1 best seller on the *New York Times* book list. This only confirms the old saying, "Given the choice of being good or being lucky, always opt for being lucky."

Of course, with this new success my two most dreaded words—*fad diet*—were immediately attached to the book. Although the word *diet* comes from the ancient Greek root meaning "way of life," it has been corrupted to imply a short-term period of hunger and deprivation to try to look good in a swimsuit. A fad is a short-term phenomenon without substance that will soon fade. Put these two words together, and you have *fad diet*. Some fad diets are simply ridiculous, such as the Drinking Man's Diet. Other fad diets, unfortunately, gain substantial credence, such as the low-fat, high-carbohydrate (rich in grains and starches) diet supported by the USDA in the early 1990s. This fad had the initial support of the government and the medical establishment, but it's clear today that this policy led to an explosion of obesity in America.

That's why I developed the concept of the Zone—not as a diet or a weight-loss program, but as a dietary road map for reaching and maintaining a constant hormonal balance that allows the body to operate at peak efficiency. The Zone is a real physiological state that can be measured in the body—a metabolic state that, once you reach it, works quickly to dramatically diminish your risk of obesity, diabetes, heart disease, and many other chronic health issues. Reaching the Zone and staying there requires a dietary lifestyle change that has to be followed for a lifetime, but it is one that will allow us to look, feel, and live healthier for many years to come.

For several years after the publication of *The Zone,* I spent my time like any good politician pressing the flesh trying to explain the mysterious world of hormones and inflammation. Now, nearly twenty years later, the once radical concept of the Zone seems almost old-fashioned, because today most diet books stress that hormones are involved in weight gain— excess insulin makes you fat and keeps you fat. Likewise, most diet books tell you if you eat too many white carbohydrates (bread, pasta, and pizza), you are going to gain weight.

But very few of today's diet books talk about inflammation as the underlying cause of why these things happen, and why it's so critical to control.

The reason the Zone concept went from being labeled a fad diet to mainstream nutrition is the science. When *The Zone* was first published, one of the few people who actually bought the book was David Ludwig, then a young Harvard Medical School instructor. (He is now a full professor at Harvard and one of the leading researchers in the study of obesity.) Actually, David first read the book with an academic's skeptical eye, concerned about pseudoscience lurking behind another fad diet. After reading the book and seeing the early scientific support (it was the first diet book to actually contain scientific references), he asked me to give a seminar to his colleagues in the division of endocrinology at Boston Children's Hospital at Harvard.

So I gave my seminar, and at the end I asked if there were any obvious fallacies to my concepts. The answer was no, since everyone seemed to be satisfied that everything I said was theoretically reasonable. Intrigued by my presentation, David decided to test my Zone concept in a controlled-feeding study. He used internal funds at Children's Hospital, because his initial attempts to get government funding for this "radical" idea were rejected.

Sure enough, David and his group found my predictions about the ability of the Zone Diet (and in particular just a single meal put together based on the Zone principles) to alter hormonal responses were true. Since then, one carefully controlled study after another has confirmed what I hypothesized twenty years ago about the power of food to control hormonal responses and reduce inflammation.

Has anything changed in my thinking about the Zone over the years? Well, yes and no. *The Zone* was the first book to describe anti-inflammatory diets and how the hormonal response to diet could either increase or decrease the levels of inflammation in the body. The Zone Diet provides a dietary blueprint for balancing food ingredients on your plate for optimal hormonal, inflammatory, and genetic control for a lifetime (as opposed to being "on a diet" and constantly hungry and fatigued in order to lose a few pounds). Nothing has changed about that basic concept. But new research continues to demonstrate just how critical it is that we act now to bring inflammation under control and how certain food ingredients can enhance the process.

Breakthroughs in molecular biology and genetics have greatly expanded our understanding of the importance of the diet in turning on and off our genes. In particular, it involves new insights in understanding how the most primitive part of our immune system responds to certain nutrients. Even more important is how our diet can further alter the expression of our genes for several generations through the new knowledge of "epigenetics." Epigenetics is like the cloud in the world of computers. It controls the expression of our genes and is strongly influenced by our environment, in particular our diet. More important, epigenetics explains how chemical markers can be left on our genes that can be amplified and transmitted to the next generation.

The Zone idea remains at the cutting edge of nutritional science because new discoveries keep adding depth to my basic concept. I first described the use of high-dose omega-3 fatty acids for anti-inflammatory control in *The OmegaRx Zone*, published in 2002. *The Mediterranean Zone* extends my basic Zone concept by describing the power of polyphenols—the chemicals that give fruits and vegetables their color—to further enhance the metabolic control of our genes and also to slow down the aging process.

The title of this book, *The Mediterranean Zone*, might suggest it will cater to those who simply want to hear that eating pasta with a little more

Parmesan cheese, drinking a little more red wine, adding some olive oil to your meals, or sipping a cappuccino with a piece of dark chocolate are the essence of the dietary program. In fact, the key feature of the diets in virtually every region that borders the Mediterranean Sea is not pasta but colorful carbohydrates rich in polyphenols. We finally have enough scientific sophistication to realize it is the high levels of colorful polyphenols that make the Mediterranean diet uniquely protective against aging, not the white pasta.

This book is divided into four parts. Part I puts the useful stuff right up front as it describes how to master the Mediterranean Zone. Part II describes the science of polyphenols. Part III describes how the industrialization of food led to an epidemic of inflammation in America that is now spreading worldwide due to globalization. Finally, Part IV describes the future that makes the concepts of the Mediterranean Zone more important than ever in reversing our current health-care crisis.

I know that after reading this book, you will agree that the continued evolution of my Zone concept is more relevant today than when it was first presented nearly twenty years ago. And with the Mediterranean Zone, it gets even more delicious!

The Zone at a Glance

The Zone is not some mystical place or a clever marketing term. It is a real physiological state in your body that can be measured in clinical tests that are routinely used at Harvard Medical School. If you are in the Zone, you have optimized your ability to control inflammation. Inflammation is the reason you gain weight, become sick, and age faster. By reducing inflammation we lose excess body fat, return to wellness, and slow the aging process.

The only way to reach the Zone and stay there for a lifetime is by your diet. The Zone Diet is not a diet but a blueprint for how to balance a meal to optimize your hormonal response for the next five hours, thus allowing you to control the levels of inflammation in your body. All you need is a hand, an eye, and a watch to follow this blueprint for life and to dramatically reduce your risk of obesity and the other major health scourges of today.

Following the Zone Diet blueprint is easy. At every meal, divide your plate into three equal sections. (You need an eye for that.) On one-third of the plate put some low-fat protein that is no larger or thicker than the palm of your hand (that's because some hands are larger than others). This doesn't have to be animal protein, but it has to be protein-rich. For vegans this means either extra-firm tofu or soy imitation-meat products. For lacto-ovo vegetarians, it can also include dairy and egg protein-rich sources in addition to vegan sources of protein. For omnivores, the choice of proteins is even wider.

To start controlling inflammation for a lifetime, just follow the figures below to start building your plate to generate an anti-inflammatory meal every time you eat.

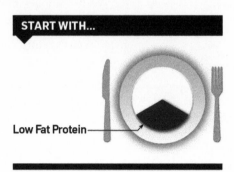

Next, fill the other two-thirds of your plate with colorful carbohydrates, primarily non-starchy vegetables and small amounts of fruits to balance the protein as shown below.

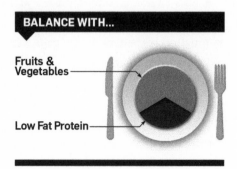

Here are two very practical hints when it comes to carbohydrates. First, the more white (white bread, white pasta, white rice, and white potatoes) you put on your plate, the more inflammation you are going to create. Second, the more non-starchy vegetables you consume and the fewer grains and starches you eat (ideally none), the better the results. Scientifically, it's called lowering the glycemic load of the meal. Finally, you add a dash of fat (a small amount). The fat I'm talking about is primarily monounsaturated fat, and low in omega-6 and saturated fats. This could be olive oil, guacamole, or nuts.

Now, why do you need the watch? If you have balanced your plate correctly, then for five hours after the meal, you will not be hungry because you have stabilized blood sugar levels. Because of those stable blood sugar levels, you will also have peak mental acuity for the same time period. The lack of hunger and improved mental focus also indicate that you have been successful in reducing inflammation in your body during that same five-hour period.

That's it. It seems easy enough, except you have to do it every five hours for the rest of your life to maintain hormonal balance and the resulting control of inflammation. That's a small price to pay for a longer and better life. And if you have a bad meal (and we all will), don't worry, since you are only one meal away from getting back into the Zone.

Since the Zone concept is simply a blueprint to balance your plate, this makes it compatible with all dietary philosophies, ranging from vegan to paleo. The balance on the plate doesn't change, only the food ingredients you use to fill in the Zone blueprint. Welcome to the Zone.

PART I

Mastering the Mediterranean Zone

1

The Coming Reckoning

Medicine is not as complicated as we are led to believe. Conversely, nutrition is not as simple as we are often told. But they are both intimately linked through inflammation.

We often think of inflammation as harmful, yet it is our primary defense in our endless struggle against microbes. Without inflammation our injuries would never heal.

Inflammation is actually a two-part process. The initial phase is an aggressive pro-inflammatory response that can turn on otherwise silent inflammatory genes to respond to injury or microbial attack. This starts with the activation of the most primitive part of our immune system to cause otherwise benign white cells in the blood to become powerful killing machines to stop the damage caused by physical injury or microbial invasion. The second phase is driven by a totally different set of protective anti-inflammatory responses, to turn off these molecular warfare mechanisms and return the body to equilibrium. Hormones ultimately determine the turning on and off of these inflammatory genes in the body.

The good news is these key hormones can be controlled by your diet. The bad news is these key hormones can become unbalanced by your diet. If these two powerful phases of inflammation are balanced, we remain in a state of wellness. If they become unbalanced, we begin a slow, steady descent into chronic disease and premature aging.

Although inflammation is a finely defined system of checks and balances that have evolved over millions of years, it can also be turned very quickly against us by our diet. Unfortunately for us, there has been a fundamental shift in the balance of these two powerful opposing inflammatory processes due to the industrialization of our food in the past fifty years, and it is only with advances in modern molecular biology that we are realizing the metabolic and genetic consequences of this change to our diet. We see this in our increased obesity, the development of chronic disease at an earlier age, and the acceleration of the aging process—especially in brain aging—and we seem to be powerless to stop them. But what if obesity, chronic disease, and aging have a common point of origin that we have overlooked?

I have spent most of my research career seeking the connections between diet and inflammation. It's a complex story that continues to rapidly evolve. But when you make a complex story too simple, the truth within the story is often the first casualty. There is no single dietary villain in this story; rather it is the complex interactions of the various changes of the American diet that have disrupted this carefully crafted balance in our inflammatory responses. More ominously, these disruptions in our inflammatory genes appear to have the ability to be transmitted and amplified from one generation to the next.

There is a coming global tsunami of the most dreaded disease of aging: Alzheimer's disease. It has been gathering strength for more than fifty years, first starting with our obesity crisis, followed by our growing diabetes epidemic, and now beginning its next manifestation as the incidence of Alzheimer's climbs.

The inflammation-to-Alzheimer's progression is shown in the following simple flow chart.

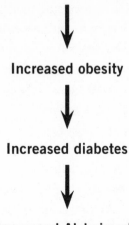

Increased diet-induced inflammation

Increased obesity

Increased diabetes

Increased Alzheimer's

It's helpful to think of this progression as a champagne fountain: It takes about fifteen to twenty years for one condition to reach a critical mass before its effects spill over into the next "bowl" and precipitate another more devastating chronic disease condition. Our obesity epidemic began to rise in the mid-1970s, but it was fueled by the beginnings of diet-induced inflammation in the early 1960s with the increasing industrialization of our food supply. The rate of diabetes was relatively constant until 1995, when it started to rise dramatically. We are now on the cusp of a new epidemic rise of Alzheimer's.

There is no known treatment to stop the progression of Alzheimer's, let alone a cure for the condition. In fact, the only thing we know about Alzheimer's is that it appears to involve inflammation. The death rates for most major diseases of the twentieth century (heart disease, cancer, stroke) have been decreasing in the past decade, but the death rate for Alzheimer's in the same period has increased by 68 percent and it is now the sixth leading cause of death in America. This suggests that as we live longer and become more inflamed by our diet, more and more of us will be victims of dementia. Not a very pleasant vision of the future.

All of these conditions—obesity, diabetes, and Alzheimer's—have a common origin: diet-induced inflammation. Keeping this type of inflammation under control means constantly keeping the hormones—generated by the food we eat—within a zone that is not too high but not too low. This is no different from taking a prescription drug. The key is keeping that drug in a therapeutic zone. If you give a patient too little of the drug, it doesn't work. If you give the patient too much of the drug, it becomes toxic. The same is true of hormones such as insulin that are critical to our metabolism and eicosanoids that control inflammation, except these hormones are hundreds of times more powerful than any drug. That was the message of *The Zone* twenty years ago, and it remains the same today. Simply stated, if you want to live a longer and better life, you have to manage diet-induced inflammation for a lifetime.

The Zone is not some mystical place. Being in the Zone is defined by rigorous clinical markers, and virtually every leading medical researcher would agree that reaching the clinical goals that define the Zone is necessary for a longer and better life. The Zone has never been an unattainable destination. However, the only way to get there is through the diet.

The Mediterranean Zone describes how we got into this health-care crisis, and it explains the potential way out of it: by following an anti-inflammatory diet that allows you to retake control of the expression of ancient inflammatory genes. If we don't do this, we can begin to prepare ourselves for World War A (A as in *Alzheimer's*).

This is why the heightened attention around traditional Mediterranean diets offers us an opportunity to retake control of our future. New advances in molecular biology and genetics now allow us to understand how certain nutrients in the Mediterranean diet can take the classic Zone Diet to an even higher level of inflammation control. In particular, it is the role of a unique group of chemicals known as polyphenols—the chemicals that give fruits and vegetables their color—to manage both the master genetic switches that control inflammation and the metabolism that offers us the greatest hope. Foods containing high levels of polyphenols have been the foundation of the Mediterranean diet for more than two thousand years and are integral dietary components for the Mediterranean Zone, which may be our best "drug" for treating obesity, chronic disease, and aging (especially in the brain) in the future.

2

Inflammation: The Real Reason We Gain Weight, Get Sick, and Age at a Faster Rate

One of great mysteries of life is how metabolism works. Food containing protein, carbohydrates, and fat (as well as vitamins, minerals, and phytochemicals) goes into our mouths, gets broken down to its most basic components for absorption, and then those components are reassembled as complex biological molecules needed to sustain life. Metabolism not only provides the continuous source of energy required for us to function, but it also allows us to continually renew every cell in our body, to defend ourselves from constant microbial invasions, repair our injuries, and finally to reproduce the next generation.

The word *metabolism* comes from the Greek root *meta*, meaning "change." That's far too simple a word to describe what actually takes place during metabolism. Metabolism can either create energy from biological matter or build complex biological molecules from simple dietary components. What is important is the fact that when your metabolism doesn't work properly, you begin to gain weight, develop chronic disease, and age at a faster rate.

Consider the complexity of trying to keep 10 trillion cells in your body in constant communication. The reason your metabolism works as smoothly as it does is because it uses a biological Internet, one vastly more complex than anyone at Google can fantasize about in the future. Unlike the simple flow of electrons that drives the computer-based Internet, your biological Internet runs on hormones, and like any good engineering system, hormones operate best when maintained within an optimal zone.

There are hundreds of known hormones (and many more still to be discovered), yet the one hormone we hear about the most is insulin and usually in negative terms. It is true that excess insulin makes you fat and keeps you fat. However, without adequate levels of this hormone much of your metabolism would grind to a halt. It is insulin that drives basic nutrients (amino acids, glucose, and fatty acids) into cells to serve as building blocks for cellular renewal or potentially as energy for the cell. It is insulin that removes what could be toxic levels of fatty acids and glucose from the bloodstream to protect your other organs. It is insulin that safely stores those excess fatty acids and glucose in the blood in your fat cells and your liver to be released at exactly the right time when we need it for energy. It is insulin that controls our hunger. It is insulin that activates key enzymes needed for growth and renewal. Yet for insulin to act as this central hub for metabolism to work its wonders, it must be maintained in a zone that is neither too high nor too low. If insulin levels are too low, your cells will starve for lack of nutrients. If insulin levels are too high, obesity, chronic disease, and accelerated aging are likely in your future.

There are two ways to increase insulin levels. One way is to eat too many carbohydrates, especially grains and starches. The other is eating too many calories. Americans have been doing both for the past forty years. Not surprisingly, as insulin levels have increased in the population, so has the incidence of obesity and other chronic diseases. But focusing on insulin alone as the agent of our current health-care demise in America is like losing your wallet and then looking for it two blocks away under a streetlamp. While there is more light under the streetlamp, you are never going to find your wallet if you just look there.

The real cause of our health-care crisis is not just carbohydrate consumption alone, but also the even more rapid rise of omega-6 fatty acids in the American diet. When *excess* omega-6 fatty acids interact with *excess* insulin, the result is the generation of molecular building blocks necessary to produce very powerful inflammatory hormones known as eicosanoids. The combination of these two recent dietary changes (increased insulin and increased omega-6 fatty acids) is like adding a lighted match to a vat of gasoline; it has resulted in an explosion of diet-induced inflammation.

We usually think of inflammation as something that hurts—you pull a muscle, then it swells and becomes inflamed (it hurts). You might consider this to be "hot" inflammation. The diet-induced inflammation I am talking about might be considered "cold" inflammation because you can't feel it. Nonetheless, this diet-induced inflammation, technically called cellular inflammation, is the type that kills. Because you can't feel it, cellular inflammation lingers for years, if not decades, until there is enough organ damage to generate chronic disease. It could be diabetes, heart disease, cancer, or even Alzheimer's. The end result is that you age before your time. To add insult to injury, cellular inflammation makes you fatter.

Diet-induced inflammation disrupts the hormonal signaling within your biological Internet, which leads to disturbances in your metabolism. The end result of altered metabolism is the development of chronic diseases at an earlier age and the acceleration of aging, especially in the brain.

The basic biochemistry of increased dietary-induced inflammation hasn't changed since I wrote my first book, *The Zone*, nearly twenty years ago. Keeping this type of inflammation in the Zone is much more difficult than simply controlling insulin (which is difficult enough). To control diet-induced inflammation for a lifetime, you have to control *both* insulin and the levels of omega-6 fatty acids. To simply reduce insulin levels without reducing omega-6 fatty acids at the same time completely misses the real cause of our current health-care problems.

The increase in diet-induced inflammation is only part of our growing epidemic of chronic disease. Remember, inflammation is a two-part process. The second component of our inflammatory response, the resolution phase, has also been under attack because of the decreased consumption of omega-3 fatty acids and polyphenols.

Each of these phases (inflammation and resolution) of the inflammatory process works independently of the other, but when they get out of sync together, you have a major metabolic disaster on your hands that accelerates virtually every known chronic disease.

Let's examine each dietary trend and how it affects the different phases of inflammation.

INCREASING OUR PRO-INFLAMMATORY RESPONSE

Increased Consumption of Omega-6 Fatty Acids

We need *some* omega-6 fatty acids to maintain a healthy ability to fight off microbes and heal from injuries. But when the levels of omega-6 fatty acids in the diet become too high, they generate excess pro-inflammatory hormones. Until recently, the levels of omega-6 fatty acids found in the human diet were very low. It is estimated that the consumption of omega-6 fatty acids in the United States has increased by more than 400 percent in the past one hundred years, with most of that increase coming in the past fifty years.

So where are these omega-6 fatty acids coming from? The answer is vegetable oils such as corn oil, soybean oil, safflower oil, sunflower oil, and others. These are now the cheapest form of calories known and they make food taste better. This is why processed foods you might eat such as fried foods, pastries (think doughnuts), and virtually everything else you find in the aisles of the supermarket are rich in omega-6 fatty acids.

In addition, omega-6 fatty acids are prone to oxidation (especially in the absence of polyphenols), which generate free radicals and other exceptionally reactive compounds that can oxidize other key players in metabolism such as lipoproteins, proteins, and DNA. These oxidation products are far more destructive to your health than any amounts of free radicals coming from UV radiation. At least you can block free radical formation from sunlight using a sunscreen. But the only way to block oxidative production coming from omega-6 fatty acids is not to eat them or at least consume very high levels of nature's most powerful anti-oxidants— polyphenols—to combat them.

Increased Consumption of High-Glycemic Carbohydrates

The industrialization of food is the primary reason for the growth of high-glycemic carbohydrates in the diet. High-glycemic carbohydrates are those that enter into the bloodstream as rapidly as glucose. Yes, these carbohydrates are in junk food, but let's not forget white bread, white pasta, white rice, and white potatoes. Sad but true, the whole-grain versions of these same carbohydrates are also high-glycemic carbohydrates. As you increase any of these foods in your diet, you will increase the secretion of the hormone insulin.

In the presence of high levels of insulin, the transformation of omega-6 fatty acids into arachidonic acid (the molecular building block of inflammatory eicosanoids) is rapidly accelerated, and cellular inflammation increases as shown below.

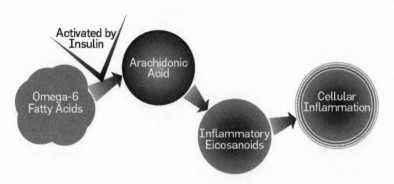

One of the consequences of increased cellular inflammation is the development of insulin resistance—the beginning stage of diabetes. Although insulin can still bind to its receptor at the cell surface, the transmission of that signal to the interior of the cell becomes compromised. Instead of being taken up by the target cells, blood glucose and fats remain elevated. As a result, the pancreas is forced to continually increase the secretion of even more insulin to help drive the excess blood glucose and fat into its target cells. This results in elevated blood insulin levels around the clock. The constantly elevated insulin levels now accelerate the further metabolism of omega-6 fatty acids into even more inflammatory eicosanoids. The result is a fast-forwarding of even more cellular inflammation. Increasing insulin resistance, caused by diet-induced inflammation, drives the metabolic complications of obesity, not simply eating carbohydrates.

DECREASING OUR ANTI-INFLAMMATORY RESOLUTION RESPONSE

Decreased Consumption of Omega-3 Fatty Acids

Humans have always had two anti-inflammatory dietary cards up their sleeves. The first of these dietary insurance policies is adequate intake of omega-3 fatty acids. Unlike pro-inflammatory omega-6 fatty acids, omega-3 fatty acids are anti-inflammatory. As long as omega-6 and omega-3 fatty acids are in balance, you maintain a healthy inflammatory response that enables you to respond to microbial invasion or injuries, but does not cause a chronic inflammatory attack on your own body. More important, omega-3 fatty acids are necessary to turn off, or resolve, the inflammatory response to allow the body to return to normal. The lack of omega-3 fatty acids in the diet is the second half of a one-two hit to your future wellness. First, you have an overreaction of an initial inflammatory response due to increased omega-6 fatty acids, and second, you can't turn it off effectively because of a lack of omega-3 fatty acids.

It is estimated that intake of omega-3 fatty acids in the American diet is only 5 to 10 percent of what it was a century ago. This is because fish (until recently) has always been an inexpensive source of protein. The more fatty fish you eat, the more anti-inflammatory omega-3 fatty acids you consume, as they are stored in the fat of the fish. Also children in the first half of the twentieth century had to take a tablespoon of cod liver oil (the world's most disgusting food) before they could leave the house. Today fatty fish consumption is down and cod liver oil is no longer standard issue in every home in America. As a result, the ratio of omega-6 to omega-3 fatty acids in Americans has increased dramatically in the last century, and again most of that increase has come in the last fifty years.

Decreased Consumption of Polyphenols

When I wrote *The Zone* in 1995, little was known about polyphenols. Today we know a lot more, including the fact that they are potent anti-inflammatory agents, but only if you consume a lot of them. High levels of polyphenols activate a genetic master switch that turns off inflammatory genes. Unfortunately, the consumption of colorful carbohydrates rich in polyphenols (fruits and vegetables) has decreased at exactly the same time that the consumption of white carbohydrates and omega-6 fatty acids has increased. The result is more cellular inflammation.

It is best to think of cellular inflammation in terms of a nuclear reactor. As you pull out the anti-inflammatory control rods (omega-3 fatty acids and polyphenols), the core of the reactor (omega-6 fatty acids and elevated insulin combining to generate more cellular inflammation) begins to heat up. If you push the anti-inflammatory control rods back into the nuclear reactor, the pro-inflammatory core cools down. Of course, if you take out the anti-inflammatory control rods completely, then you get a meltdown of the reactor. This is what has been happening in America for the past fifty years.

So there you have it. There is no single "evil one," such as fructose, milk, or wheat (more about these dietary mythologies later), but a combination of factors that are putting us at high risk of increased cellular inflammation and a resulting lifetime of misery. This is why our current epidemics of obesity and diabetes seem to have appeared out of nowhere and why we seem powerless to reverse them.

The role of inflammation in weight gain, development of chronic disease, and aging is complex. The following will give you a short overview that you can explore in greater detail in the Appendices.

How We Get Fat

Although the diet book industry is devoted to weight loss, no one seems to describe how we actually get fat. I will describe the actual process in greater detail in the Appendices, but let me summarize it here.

It is true that excess insulin makes you fat and keeps you fat. However, excess insulin is not caused by lack of willpower, but by the disruption of your fat metabolism by cellular inflammation. Under ideal conditions, fat gets taken up from the blood and is stored in your fat cells to be released at a later time (such as when you are sleeping) to supply energy for the rest of your body. The levels of insulin in the blood control this process. When you develop insulin resistance, this careful balance of fat uptake and fat release is disrupted. The end result is that you get fatter as fat from the bloodstream is accumulated more readily by your fat cells and cannot be as easily used as fuel by other cells. Carbohydrates alone don't make you fat; it is the diet-induced inflammation they contribute to in the presence of excess omega-6 fatty acids that makes you fat.

How We Get Sick

Many of our chronic diseases can be viewed as disturbances in metabolism. These include diabetes and heart disease. Other chronic diseases, such as autoimmune disorders (arthritis, lupus, multiple sclerosis, asthma, allergies, and so on), are a consequence of increased cellular inflammation, and many neurological disorders (ADHD, depression, Parkinson's, Alzheimer's, and so on) and cancer may be viewed as a combination of both.

As you increase cellular inflammation, the necessary hormonal signaling that is required for a stable metabolism is disrupted. Increased cellular inflammation also activates the most primitive part of the immune system to mount a continuing attack mode. Eventually this leads to organ malfunction, and we call that chronic disease.

Why the Rate of Aging (Especially in the Brain) Is Increasing

As increased cellular inflammation interferes with your body's ability to signal metabolic disruptions, your organs begin to operate less efficiently. That's when the physical signs of aging (increased body fat, loss of muscle mass, increased fatigue, development of wrinkles, and so on) begin to appear. Not surprisingly, the practice of "anti-aging" medicine usually depends on increasing certain hormone levels in the body. However, this doesn't overcome the primary underlying problem, which is the disturbance of hormonal signaling caused by increased cellular inflammation. Solve that problem by following an anti-inflammatory diet, and you will do a lot more to reduce the real rate of aging inside your cells than any amount of hormone supplementation.

Far more ominous to your future is the increasing likelihood of developing dementia, especially in the form of Alzheimer's disease. It is estimated that, in America, one-third of individuals older than age 65 will die with some form of dementia. Alzheimer's disease itself is the fifth leading cause of death of individuals older than age 65. By the time a person reaches age 85, approximately 50 percent will have some form of Alzheimer's. If you have diabetes, you are twice as likely to develop Alzheimer's.

That's why many neurologists are beginning to call Alzheimer's disease type 3 diabetes. What they should be saying is that both diabetes and Alzheimer's are diseases of inflammation. In diabetes, the pancreas is inflamed. In Alzheimer's, the brain is inflamed. The earlier you develop type 2 diabetes and the longer its duration, the greater the risk of developing Alzheimer's. This means we may have a neurological tsunami awaiting us in a very short period of time. The treatment of dementia has already become one of the most costly drains on our health-care system and will only continue to grow as the current generation ages.

Not a very pretty picture for the future of America (as well as the rest of the world). Humans will become fatter, sicker, and demented, primarily due to increased diet-induced inflammation. Fortunately, the next chapter provides a dietary road map to begin to reverse those consequences.

3

Mastering the Zone Diet
for a Lifetime

If your goal is to lose weight and improve health, then the only way to get there is to reduce diet-induced inflammation. The Mediterranean Zone is your road map.

Reaching the Zone will reduce inflammation by keeping insulin, eicosanoids, and other food-generated hormones within therapeutic ranges twenty-four hours a day, so you are always moving toward optimum health through hormonal balance. Although that may sound intimidating, it really is not. To enter the Zone you need only three things, which you probably have with you wherever you go: a hand, an eye, and a watch. If you have those tools, then a lifetime living in the Zone—perfectly in balance and at dramatically lowered risk for weight gain, diabetes, Alzheimer's, and other modern scourges—becomes incredibly easy.

Every meal (and that includes breakfast) starts with a plate. Now use your eye to divide the plate into three equal parts. On one-third of the plate, add some low-fat protein such as chicken or fish, or even vegetarian protein-rich products such as extra-firm tofu or soybean imitation-meat substitutes. Just make sure the protein portion on the plate is no larger or thicker than the palm of your hand. This is about 3 ounces of low-fat protein for the average female and about 4 ounces of low-fat protein for the average male This is the standard recommendation among most registered dieticians. I would agree with them that you should never exceed that amount of protein at a meal.

Next, fill the rest of the plate with colorful, low-glycemic load carbohydrates, such as vegetables and fruits. Bright colors signal that they are rich in polyphenols, which help to control diet-induced inflammation. Nonstarchy vegetables (broccoli, peppers, onions, asparagus, and so on) are the best sources of carbohydrates since they have a very low glycemic load. This means they don't generate a large insulin response when eaten, even though they take up a lot of room on the plate. Fruits have a higher glycemic load, and whole grains have a very high glycemic load. White carbohydrates (bread, pasta, rice, and potatoes) simply have no place on your Zone plate because of their high glycemic load and lack of polyphenols.

Finally, add a little (that means a dash of) fat that is low in both omega-6 and saturated fatty acids. For most people, the best choice is extra-virgin olive oil.

So that covers the eye and the hand. But why do you need the watch? If you created the right balance of protein, carbohydrates, and fat for that particular meal, then for the next five hours you won't be hungry, and you will maintain peak mental focus and emotional balance because you have stabilized blood glucose levels.

The reasons that this dietary blueprint gets you to the Zone are as follows:

1. Your hormonal control is based on the balance of protein to glycemic load at every meal.

You don't get to "bank" this hormonal control, as it will last only about five hours. The best thing about the Mediterranean Zone is that a correctly balanced meal will bring you into the Zone and start reducing inflammation immediately, no matter what your nutritional past may have been. But even with a perfectly balanced Zone meal, the hormonal changes will last only five hours. This means you are hormonally only as good as your last meal.

So to optimize your health and weight loss, you have to pay attention to the balance of protein to the glycemic load at every meal. Technically the glycemic load is defined as the total of the individual amounts of each carbohydrate on the plate multiplied by their individual glycemic responses (the glycemic index). What the glycemic load provides you is an indication of how rapidly your blood glucose levels will rise after a meal. The lower the glycemic load of a meal, the less insulin you produce for the next five hours. If you eat a lot of grains (even whole grains) and starches, blood glucose rises quickly after a meal; so then do your insulin levels, as insulin is secreted to reduce that sudden influx of glucose into the blood. If you replace the grains with fruit (not fruit juices), legumes, and especially non-starchy vegetables, blood glucose levels don't rise as quickly—and insulin response remains modest.

The more rapid the rise of blood glucose levels, the greater the secretion of insulin to reduce those levels in the blood. The insulin (1) causes the storage of excess glucose either in the liver or muscles (as glycogen), (2) converts excess glucose into fatty acids in the liver that are released into the blood, and (3) helps convert some excess glucose to glycerol and enhances the transport of fatty acids into the fat cells—which then helps transfer excess fatty acids from your blood to your adipose tissue, where fatty acids can be safely stored.

The reason the body produces insulin rapidly in response to elevated blood glucose levels is that, in excess, glucose is toxic. It reacts with protein in the blood to form advanced glycosylated end (AGE) products. These "sugar-coated" proteins can bind to specific receptors (called RAGE, or receptors for advanced glycosylated end products) in your cells that initiate inflammatory responses. One of the consequences of increased inflammation is the development of insulin resistance, a condition that results in chronically elevated insulin levels. This is the real reason insulin makes you fat and keeps you fat.

And it's also the reason reducing the glycemic load of your meals is so important. Protein belongs on your plate to promote satiety and to stimulate the release of hormones that stabilize blood sugar levels. The secret to the success of the Zone Diet is that you are never hungry (because satiety is increased) and never fatigued (because blood glucose levels are stabilized).

2. The real danger of the current American diet is the deadly combination of excess omega-6 fatty acids coupled with high levels of insulin.

The continuing consumption of omega-6 fatty acids (primarily from vegetable oils such as soybean, corn, sunflower, and safflower) combined with high-glycemic carbohydrates (refined carbohydrates, whole-grain carbohydrates, and white starches such as potatoes and rice) sets the stage for increased levels of diet-induced inflammation by enhancing the synthesis of arachidonic acid (the driver of cellular inflammation). Arachidonic acid (AA) is the driver of cellular inflammation because it is the molecular building block for powerful pro-inflammatory eicosanoids. You might consider AA to be toxic fat, far more dangerous to your health than any trans fat or saturated fat could possibly be. High concentrations of AA can be found in egg yolks and organ meats. However, AA can come from omega-6 fatty acids (primarily in vegetable oils) and a high-glycemic-load diet. The increased secretion of insulin (induced by the rapid entry of glucose into the bloodstream) will accelerate the conversion of omega-6 fatty acids into AA. It is like adding a lighted match to a vat of gasoline. It's a deadly combination as you get an explosion of cellular inflammation. Why deadly? Cellular inflammation accelerates the development of chronic disease and speeds up the aging process by disrupting hormonal signaling patterns in every cell. This is the real reason you get fatter, become sicker, and age faster.

3. Excess omega-6 fatty acids also increase oxidation throughout the body—unless you have adequate levels of polyphenols in the diet.

You have a hot body—about 98.6 degrees Fahrenheit, in fact—and it's exposed twenty-four hours a day to high levels of oxygen. As you know from storing fruit on the counter in summer, heat plus oxygen leads to spoilage. When the same happens to lipids, you call it rancidity. And that's exactly what happens to the omega-6 fatty acids you consume—they become rancid inside the body. These oxidized fats not only cause inflammation but also can accelerate heart disease by creating oxidized LDL particles (the *really* bad cholesterol).

This is exactly why the Mediterranean Zone is so effective in fighting disease. Polyphenols—which are powerful antioxidants (far more than vitamin E or vitamin C)—are found in high levels in the colorful carbohydrates (vegetables and fruits) that are the primary carbohydrates of the Mediterranean diet and of the Mediterranean Zone. Of course, it makes even better dietary sense to reduce omega-6 fatty acids and increase polyphenols at the same time.

4. Lack of adequate levels of omega-3 fatty acids and polyphenols make it difficult to control diet-induced inflammation.

Unlike omega-6 fatty acids, the long-chain omega-3 fatty acids found in fish and fish oils are anti-inflammatory. Polyphenols in high enough levels are also anti-inflammatory. If you don't have adequate levels of both in your diet, your ability to turn off inflammation is highly compromised.

Control these separate dietary changes—properly balanced protein and low-glycemic carbohydrates, significantly reduced intake of omega-6 fatty acids, and significantly increased intake of polyphenols and omega-3 fatty acids—and you will always be inside the Zone where the control of cellular inflammation induced by the diet can be maintained for a lifetime. By reducing diet-induced inflammation, you will also lose excess body fat, decrease the likelihood of developing chronic disease, and slow down the aging process. Your body will become more adept at converting food calories to chemical energy. And because you are reducing cellular inflammation, the hormonal signals that tell the brain to stop eating become more effective. As a result, you will not be hungry.

If you aren't hungry, then you consume fewer calories. Consume fewer calories without hunger and fatigue, and you will lose excess body fat, delay the development of chronic disease, and live longer. That is the secret of the Mediterranean Zone.

If you want to be more technical, these simple rules result in a calorie distribution that is about 40 percent low-glycemic-load carbohydrates (primarily non-starchy vegetables), 30 percent low-fat protein (such as chicken, fish, or tofu and soy imitation-meat products), and 30 percent fat (mostly monounsaturated fat, and low in both omega-6 and saturated fats).

I prefer to keep the total carbohydrate intake at about 40 percent of your calories because the brain is literally a glucose hog. The brain accounts for only 2 percent of the mass of the total body, but it uses 20 percent of the blood glucose. The brain requires about 130 grams of glucose per day, which is why the Mediterranean Zone provides between 100 and 150 grams of carbohydrates per day, split over three meals and one or two snacks. This may sound like a lot, but in fact it's about a 50 to 67 percent reduction of the total carbohydrates most Americans are currently eating.

But one must be careful to spread those carbohydrates throughout the day. Consuming more than 30 to 40 grams of carbohydrates at any one meal is going to generate excess insulin. If you are not getting five hours of appetite suppression or you feel you have reached a weight plateau, before you think about lowering the levels of carbohydrates in your diet, first begin to reduce the glycemic load of your meals. Begin by eliminating grains and starches from your diet. If this isn't sufficient to have the desired result, then start removing fruits and legumes (moderate-glycemic load carbohydrates) from your diet. This will leave non-starchy, low-glycemic load vegetables as your primary carbohydrate source. You will have a very difficult time eating enough non-starchy vegetables to overstimulate insulin, but you will still be maintaining adequate blood glucose for the brain.

A common misconception about the Zone is that it is a high-protein diet. That's simply not true. Let's look at the number of grams of macronutrients (carbohydrates, protein, and fat) a normal female or male might be consuming following the Mediterranean Zone.

Macronutrient	1,200 calories a day	1,500 calories a day
Carbohydrate	120 g/day	150 g/day
Protein	90 g/day	112 g/day
Fat	40 g/day	50 g/day

Your first thought might be, "I will starve to death on 1,200 to 1,500 calories per day." I guarantee you will not. This is what I call the Zone Paradox: You will consume fewer calories with less hunger but more energy. Furthermore, you are still eating the typical protein intake of most Americans. Even though you are consuming fewer carbohydrates (but more of the colorful, non-starchy kind), they are still the primary source of calories in the Zone Diet. Since you always are consuming more grams of carbohydrate than protein, you can't really describe the Zone as a high-protein, low-carbohydrate diet unless my definitions of high and low are significantly different from what is in the dictionary. Probably the best way to describe the Zone is as a moderate-protein, low-glycemic load diet.

Can you become too thin on the Mediterranean Zone? When you can see your abdominal muscles, it is time to start thinking about adding some additional monounsaturated fat (extra-virgin olive oil or almonds) to your diet. (So besides requiring a watch, you also might need a mirror to see if you are developing a six-pack.) This is what I do with the elite athletes (such as the twenty-five gold medal winners in the last five Olympics) who follow the Zone. Their goal is optimal performance, not being on the cover of *Men's Fitness*, and athletic performance depends on having a certain level of body fat. That fat provides the high-octane fuel needed for making the chemical energy needed for optimal performance.

The macronutrient balance of the Zone is not set in stone but represents a bell-shaped curve.

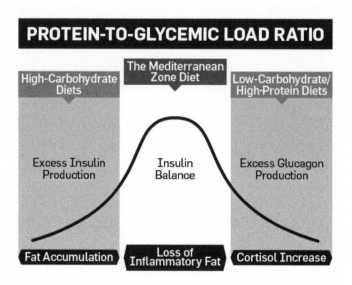

Why? Not everyone is genetically the same. Nonetheless, the more you increase carbohydrate intake (even adding moderate-glycemic ones such as fruits), the more you will increase insulin secretion. If that is combined with high amounts of omega-6 fatty acids in your diet, then you are going to create more inflammatory eicosanoids and more cellular inflammation. That's going to make you fat, sick, and age faster. If you swing too much in the other direction and have too much protein and not enough carbohydrates (such as on the Atkins diet), you are going to cause the increased secretion of cortisol, which is a stress hormone. That hormone will make you fat, sick, and age faster.

So it is critical that you keep experimenting with the balance of food ingredients on your plate until you can maintain yourself in the Zone. How do you know when you get there? Use your watch. If you can go for five hours between meals without being hungry or losing peak mental focus, that's your sign that your last meal put you into the Zone. The secret is keeping yourself in that Zone for a lifetime. The better you play this hormonal balancing game using the Mediterranean Zone, the better and easier your life becomes.

The balance of protein, carbohydrates, and fat in the Mediterranean Zone is continually reinforced by ongoing research that has been published over the last fifteen years. The dietary recommendations of the Joslin Diabetes Center at Harvard Medical School for treating obesity and diabetes are essentially those of the Mediterranean Zone. Some of the more recent research comes from the EPIC study published in 2013 analyzing the diets of some twenty-two thousand Greeks, demonstrating those following a low-glycemic load diet with a total carbohydrate intake of about 40 percent of total calories had the least risk in developing diabetes. A 2010 *British Journal of Nutrition* article estimated the diet composition of our Paleolithic ancestors was about 40 percent low-glycemic load carbohydrates, 30 percent protein, and 30 percent fat. It appears that health in the past, present, and future depends on having a balance of macronutrients. As soon as you start increasing one macronutrient in a diet, another has to decrease. Moving away from the basic Zone macronutrient balance creates very large hormonal changes that can disrupt your metabolism.

The most important research, however, is that which demonstrates the effectiveness of the Zone diet in reducing cellular inflammation. The published research leaves little doubt on this subject. Harvard Medical School demonstrated in 2004 that the Zone diet was nine times more effective in reducing inflammation compared to a control diet based on the USDA dietary recommendations, even though the weight loss was the same with both diets. Tufts University School of Medicine came to the same conclusion when comparing the Zone to the USDA dietary recommendations in treating diabetics. A study published in 2006 in the *American Journal of Clinical Nutrition* indicated that the Zone dramatically reduced cellular inflammation while simultaneously improving exercise endurance and mood levels when compared to the Atkins diet.

The reduction of diet-induced inflammation should be the real goal of any nutrition plan, as opposed to simple weight loss. It is only with the reduction of cellular inflammation that you begin to reverse chronic disease and slow down the aging process. Unfortunately, weight loss is not a good marker. This is because weight loss is made up of water loss, loss of muscle mass, and loss of excess body fat. Losing water and muscle is not going to have any positive health benefits. However, losing excess body fat does because of its reduction of inflammation. In this regard, the Zone is the clear winner.

WHAT TO EXPECT FOLLOWING THE
MEDITERRANEAN ZONE

The power of science is that it helps predict the future. If you throw a rock into the air, you can be confident it will fall back to earth. That's why gravity represents such strong science. Likewise, nutrition predictions have to come true if it is good science.

So here is what you can expect if you follow the Mediterranean Zone for a month.

1. By days 2 to 3 your hunger will be significantly decreased because you are maintaining stable blood glucose levels from meal to meal. With that stabilization of blood glucose levels comes better mental acuity and emotional stability.
2. By days 3 to 4 you will begin to experience a significant improvement in your levels of physical energy, as you are better able to access your stored body fat for the production of the chemical energy needed to move around.
3. By day 7 you will not have lost a lot of weight (it's difficult to lose more than one pound of fat per week), but your clothes will be fitting better because the weight you are losing is primarily body fat, specifically visceral body fat in your midsection. That's why your clothes are fitting better.
4. By day 14 your ability to handle stress will be significantly enhanced as cortisol levels are reduced.
5. By day 30 you will see significant changes in your blood chemistry as markers of improved health and a slowing of the aging process.

If you like that list of benefits and want to maintain them, then just continue the Mediterranean Zone for a lifetime. If you have a hand, an eye, and a watch, that's easy to do.

CLINICAL MARKERS OF THE ZONE

Ultimately nutrition has to be treated as science. So what are some of those clinical markers that are indicative of being in the Zone? Although I will discuss these markers in greater detail in Appendix E, here is a quick summary.

Blood Marker	What It Measures
AA/EPA ratio	Control of cellular inflammation
Glycosylated Hemoglobin (HbA$_1$c)	Control of blood sugar
TG/HDL ratio	Control of liver insulin resistance

Two of these tests (HbA$_1$c and TG/HDL) will usually come from blood-work issued for your annual physical. The AA/EPA ratio is a more specialized test used routinely in medical research, but not in standard blood tests given by your physician. See Appendix F for resources that will do such testing using only a drop of blood coming from a finger stick (similar to testing for blood glucose). Once you have these test numbers, you can tell if you are in the Zone, close to the Zone, or need lots of work to get to the Zone using the following chart.

Parameter	In the Zone	Close to the Zone	Needs Lots of Work
AA/EPA ratio	1.5–3	6	>10
HgA$_1$c	5%	5.5%	>6%
TG/HDL ratio	<1	2	>3

This is not a multiple-choice test. Either all three clinical markers are in the correct ranges, or you can't be considered healthy no matter how good you look in a swimsuit. Getting into the Zone remains the best medicine if your goal is the reduction of cellular inflammation leading to the reversal of chronic disease and better quality of life. Following the Mediterranean Zone is the easiest way to get to the Zone.

So what percentage of Americans might currently be in the Zone based on these clinical markers? The best evidence indicates less than 1 percent. Maybe 4 percent of the U.S. population is close to the Zone, and definitely more than 95 percent of Americans are out of the Zone by eating in a way that is increasing their chances of chronic disease and premature death. Is it any wonder that health-care costs are out of control?

I really don't care what diet you follow as long as you are never hungry for five hours after every meal, and your blood markers indicate you are in the Zone. However, if you follow my simple dietary rules, you are quite likely to feel the effects of improved hormonal control with your first meal, and within thirty days those blood markers that define the Zone will start to change for the better. Stay in the Zone for a lifetime, and you have your best chance of a longer and healthier life.

4

The Mediterranean Diet:
Facts and Fiction

Today we hear a lot about the Mediterranean diet. UNESCO, the cultural arm of the United Nations, has proclaimed the Mediterranean diet one of civilization's great treasures.

But which Mediterranean diet? There are sixteen countries that border the Mediterranean Sea. I have been to most of them for extended periods of time, and I can tell you that there is no single Mediterranean diet. What is eaten in Spain is very different from that eaten in Italy, and what is consumed in Italy is distinct from the diet in Greece, not to mention the other thirteen countries in the region.

If you ask most Americans for their definition of the Mediterranean diet, the response is usually eating pasta (and pizza), drinking red wine, using a little olive oil, drinking espresso, and adding some Parmesan cheese to their meals. But that American version doesn't look anything like the real Mediterranean diet.

The distinguishing feature of the diets in virtually every region that borders the Mediterranean Sea is not pasta but vegetables and fruits (colorful carbohydrates rich in polyphenols). We finally have enough scientific sophistication to realize that the high levels of polyphenols make the Mediterranean diet unique.

There is no definitive caloric composition that makes up the Mediterranean diet. The best that researchers can do is to estimate adherence of their subjects in the consumption of those food groups they think should be in the Mediterranean diet. These food groups include separate categories such as vegetables, fruits and nuts, legumes, olive oil, fish, and cereals (bread, pasta, rice, and so on), drinking red wine, and not eating much meat or dairy products. Based on this definition, a good guess might be that about 60 percent of the calories in the Mediterranean diet are consumed as carbohydrates, 15 percent as protein, and about 35 percent as fat, which would make the Mediterranean diet close in macronutrient composition to the current American diet. So why is it seemingly so much healthier? It's the polyphenols.

If you look at the Mediterranean food groups carefully, they usually fall into two broad categories: those rich in polyphenols (fruits, vegetables, wine) eaten in large quantities and those, such as red meat, chicken, and eggs, that are not great sources of polyphenols—and are eaten far less frequently. Furthermore, it is implicit that the fat in the Mediterranean diet is generally rich in monounsaturated fats (from olive oil and nuts), moderate in omega-3 fats (coming from fish), and low in omega-6 and saturated fats (from corn oil and red meat). Foods rich in polyphenols, monounsaturated fats, and omega-3 fatty acids and low in omega-6 and saturated fats may well explain why, despite having a similar ratio of carbohydrates, protein, and fat as the current American diet, the Mediterranean diet is so much more effective at preventing disease and promoting longevity.

Most of the research around the Mediterranean diet comes from epidemiological studies, which observe large groups of individuals to determine whether those more closely adhering to a dietary ingredient regimen have any improved health outcomes over those who are not. Better adherence to a Mediterranean diet (meaning probably eating more polyphenols) appears to reduce the incidence of diabetes and heart disease. Just as important, adherence to the Mediterranean diet also appears to preserve the mind and slow the rate of aging. Since diabetes, heart disease, and dementia are caused by cellular inflammation, this would strongly suggest that a Mediterranean diet really is an anti-inflammatory diet. However, remember that these benefits only come from a lifetime of eating a Mediterranean diet, reinforcing the ancient Greek origins of the word *diet,* which means "way of life."

Unfortunately, while longevity and a lower risk of disease are among the benefits of a traditional Mediterranean diet, weight loss is not. The Mediterranean diet is still overloaded with carbohydrates; it still falls outside the dietary composition needed to reach the Zone. If you are eating too many carbohydrates (even if they are rich in polyphenols), and they are not balanced with low-fat protein, then you are not going to lose weight. That's why I believe this book to be so essential. It's the first time the longevity-enhancing science behind the Mediterranean diet has been further enhanced by the weight-loss and anti-inflammatory power gained when you reach the Zone.

Are there any intervention studies that suggest that the Mediterranean diet has health benefits compared to a control diet, such as the diet recommended by the American Heart Association? Actually there are. The results of the first of such studies, the Lyon Diet Heart Study, didn't make the American Heart Association very happy. Started in 1988, this study split more than six hundred French patients who had recently suffered a heart attack into two groups. One group followed the American Heart Association diet guidelines, consisting of a low-saturated-fat, low-cholesterol diet, but the fat they did consume was relatively rich in omega-6 fatty acids (beloved by the AHA because they are shown to lower blood cholesterol). The other group followed an experimental diet similar to the Mediterranean diet, which included more fish, vegetables, and fruits and was low in omega-6 fatty acids. The researchers wanted their subjects to use olive oil. But because the French tend to prefer butter over olive oil, the researchers gave the subjects free margarine low in omega-6 fatty acids, but enriched with omega-3 fats and lots of trans fatty acids to hold it together. Trans fats!

They planned to follow the patients in both groups for the next five years, but the study was stopped after three and half years. Was it ended because those getting the experimental Mediterranean diet were dying like flies because of the trans fats in their diet? No, just the opposite. They were doing dramatically better (especially in terms of mortality) than the subjects following the American Heart Association recommendations. How much better? They had 70 percent fewer deaths overall and a complete elimination of sudden cardiac death (the primary reason you die from heart attack).

When researchers looked for clinical markers to explain these remarkable differences in mortality, they found the blood cholesterol levels were the same in the two groups, as were the blood sugar and blood pressure levels. The only thing they found that was different was that those following the experimental Mediterranean diet had a 30 percent lower AA/EPA ratio in their blood. Since the AA/EPA ratio is one of the markers of cellular inflammation used to define the Zone, this would also suggest that the mortality differences may be a result of reductions in cellular inflammation and not the usual suspects such as elevated cholesterol and blood pressure.

Another recently published intervention study supposedly demonstrated the superiority of the traditional Mediterranean diet compared to a low-fat diet to prevent heart disease. This study was noble in design but flawed in execution (this is the continuing story of diet intervention studies). The researchers split the subjects into three separate groups. One group was given free nuts, including walnuts and almonds. The second group was given free extra-virgin olive oil. The third was told to change their current diet to a low-fat diet. Not surprisingly, the groups that got the free food eagerly consumed it. Since the free food consisted of items that increased their adherence to the Mediterranean way of eating, it was not surprising that their Mediterranean diet adherence scores also increased. And the group that was supposed to change their diet to a low-fat diet? They didn't. So in the end the study compared people getting free food rich in polyphenols to a group that made virtually no changes to their current diet. Some controlled study! At the end of the study, those subjects getting either free nuts or free olive oil (foods rich in polyphenols) had fewer heart attacks. The media screamed this proved the Mediterranean diet prevents heart disease, when it really proved that people who consume free food rich in polyphenols seem to have fewer heart attacks. It also proved that it's very difficult to change a person's dietary habit if they don't get free food.

Other more controlled intervention studies have indicated when you dramatically reduce the levels of carbohydrates in the Mediterranean diet (usually around 60 percent total calories) and simultaneously increase the protein content from about 15 percent of total calories to about 30 percent, there are significant improvements in blood sugar control and satiety. This would suggest that there is a lot of potential improvement in what is considered to be the Mediterranean diet.

The logical question might be this: Can the benefits of the Mediterranean diet (decreased chronic disease, increased longevity, and decreased dementia) be taken to a still higher level using the Zone blueprint of balancing protein, carbohydrate, and fat in addition to providing the missing Holy Grail of weight loss at the same time?

The answer is an absolute yes, as I will explain in the next chapter.

5

The Mediterranean Zone: The Evolution of the Mediterranean Diet

If you take the composition of the Zone Diet that I described earlier and put it into a graphic form, it looks something like this:

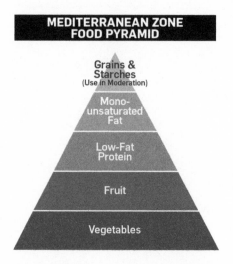

MEDITERRANEAN ZONE FOOD PYRAMID

Grains & Starches
(Use in Moderation)

Mono-unsaturated Fat

Low-Fat Protein

Fruit

Vegetables

The basis of your diet is a lot of non-starchy colorful vegetables with limited amounts of colorful fruits and legumes. You add moderate amounts of low-fat protein (such as chicken or fish) and a bit of monounsaturated fat, such as extra-virgin olive oil or limited amounts of nuts, and keep the intake of omega-6 and saturated fats to a minimum. Finally, you eat as few grains and starches as possible (zero would be the optimum) and never put any white carbohydrates on the plate. Up to this point the Mediterranean Zone seems similar to the Mediterranean diet except for the reduction or elimination of grains and starches and adding far more colorful vegetables and fruits to your plate. But those two seemingly small dietary changes have dramatic hormonal implications. It turns a good diet (the Mediterranean diet) into a hormonally superior anti-inflammatory diet (the Mediterranean Zone). To get even better results, you keep reducing the levels of the fruits and increasing the levels of non-starchy vegetables. This significantly reduces the glycemic load of the diet and further enhances its anti-inflammatory performance.

The key to the Mediterranean Zone is keeping your body in constant hormonal balance using food ingredients primarily found in the Mediterranean region. You do this with the understanding of how those food ingredients can interact hormonally and genetically to reduce diet-induced inflammation.

Unlike the relatively unstructured dietary parameters of the Mediterranean diet, the Mediterranean Zone provides a defined structure, and that is the key to generating superior results. Since the primary benefits of the traditional Mediterranean diet are better cognition and a longer life, then what can you expect by following the Mediterranean Zone? You will be smarter, happier, live a longer life with better health, and, unlike the results with the Mediterranean diet, you will also lose weight. Not a bad deal.

I've already talked in general terms about the balance of the foods that should fill your plate, but what food ingredients should you eat on the Mediterranean Zone? Let me give you a short historical overview of the changes that have taken place in the foods of the Mediterranean region, and this will give you some clues about how to make the Mediterranean Zone work optimally for you.

A. Pre-agricultural (Paleolithic) Mediterranean Ingredients

Protein-based foods during this era would have included eggs, fish, and red meat from wild game. The only carbohydrates consumed were fruits and vegetables (although cross-breeding and hybridization have changed these plants substantially since then), and the only fats were nuts, or organs (such as the brain) from wild game. Fish, vegetables, fruits, and nuts are still mainstays of the Mediterranean diet regardless of how it is defined.

B. Pre-Christianity Mediterranean Ingredients

The advent of agriculture introduced new types of carbohydrates into the Mediterranean diet, including whole grains. There was a greater variety of protein sources available then, including dairy, legumes, and poultry, as well as new sources of fat, such as olive oil, that were rich in polyphenols. Also biotechnology (that is, fermentation) was being used to make foods such as yogurt and garum (a fermented sauce from fish intestines that was the ketchup of Roman times). Of course, the biggest breakthrough in biotechnology during this time period was the discovery and development of wine, produced by the yeast-mediated fermentation of the carbohydrates in the grapes. The alcohol produced by the fermentation extracted even greater amounts of polyphenols from grape skins. Many of these biotechnology-generated foods (except for garum) still remain in the Mediterranean diet.

C. Post-Christianity Mediterranean Ingredients

The next infusion of new ingredients came during medieval times. Although urban legend has Marco Polo bringing pasta back to Italy from China, various forms of crude pasta already existed in Italy before his journey. The discovery of the Americas brought tomatoes, potatoes, and chocolate into the Mediterranean diet. Coffee came from Arabia. While tomatoes, unsweetened chocolate, and coffee are all rich in polyphenols, white potatoes are not.

And let's not forgot the introduction of refined alcohol thanks to the Benedictine monks, who learned how to distill wine to increase its alcohol content. Unfortunately, this removed the vast majority of polyphenols from the wine during the distillation process.

D. Modern Industrial Ingredients

The newest additions to the Mediterranean diet come from the new refining technologies, which both increase the shelf life of food and also reduce its cost. These include refined carbohydrates, devoid of polyphenols, such as white pasta, white bread, and white rice in addition to refined white sugar.

Another American import is refined vegetable oil (primarily corn and soy), rich in omega-6 fats. These fats were virtually unknown in all human diets until the last one hundred years. Finally, more advanced biotechnologies provided trans fats, derived from refined vegetable oils, and high-fructose corn syrup that was even cheaper than refined sugar. The last two food ingredients, coupled with cheap refined carbohydrates, became the backbone of the processed food industry.

It doesn't take a rocket (or even a nutritional) scientist to quickly figure out that the more you stick with food ingredients used in the Paleolithic and pre-Christianity Mediterranean times, the better you are going to control diet-induced inflammation as well as lose weight. As soon as you add more of the post-Christianity and the modern industrial ingredients to the diet, your chances of reaching the Zone tumble dramatically as you increase the levels of diet-induced inflammation.

A Day in the Mediterranean Zone

The key to maintaining the health benefits of the Mediterranean Zone is controlling cellular inflammation. Since the hormonal effects of a meal last only about five hours, this means you are eating about five times per day: three Mediterranean Zone meals and two Mediterranean Zone snacks. The secret is to never let more than five hours go by without an appropriate balanced meal or snack. For example, you should always consume a Mediterranean Zone meal within one hour after waking. Breakfast is the most important meal of the day because your body is on empty due to overnight fasting. If you eat breakfast at 7 a.m., this means you should have your next meal no later than noon. Since most Americans eat dinner around 7 p.m., that's more than five hours from lunch. So in the late afternoon, have a Mediterranean Zone snack to keep your hormones in the Zone until dinner. Finally, before you go to bed, have another Mediterranean Zone snack. Even though you are going to sleep, your brain isn't, and this late-night snack provides the hormonal touch-up you need so you aren't groping for that cup of coffee the next morning to try to get you started.

The beauty of the Mediterranean Zone is that there is no guilt. If you mess up with one meal that takes you out of the Zone, your next meal can put you right back where you want to be hormonally.

	DAY 1	DAY 2	DAY 3
BREAKFAST	Ham Omelet with Fruit	Vegetable Omelet with Peanut Butter Crackers	Yogurt and Berries
LUNCH	Balsamic Pork Filet over Red Onions	Beef and Broccoli	Brussels Sprouts with Warm Goat Cheese
SNACK	Blueberry Ricotta Snack	Bell Pepper and Hummus Snack	Ham and Apple Snack
DINNER	Chicken Breast in Spring Sauce	Grilled Sea Bass with Garlic Artichokes	Lamb with Eggplant and Leek Salad
SNACK	Deviled Eggs with Hummus	Quick Applesauce Snack	Turkey-Apple Crunch for Two

A WEEK IN THE MEDITERRANEAN ZONE

The Mediterranean Zone is a foolproof plan for optimal health. As long as your plate is two-thirds full of brightly colored (non-starchy) vegetables and the remaining third is made up of lean protein, you're following the Mediterranean Zone.

For those of you who would like a structured plan to start off, I have put together a week of easy-to-prepare, polyphenol-rich sample meals and snacks that are inspired by authentic Mediterranean recipes.

DAY 4	DAY 5	DAY 6	DAY 7
Salty Mousse	Spinach Omelet with Fruit Bowl	Fruit Mousse	Ham and Strawberry Cream Cheese Crackers
Roasted Vegetables with Melted Mozzarella	Orange Grilled Salmon with Fennel Tomato Salad	Shrimp Salad with Green Beans, Hearts of Palm, and Tomatoes	Orange-Vanilla Halibut with Onions and Artichoke Hearts
Pear and Parmesan Cheese Snack	Berries and Yogurt	Chocolate Mousse Snack	Whey Blueberry Snack
Chicken with Mushrooms and Peppers	Turkey with Sautéed Zucchini	Veal in Mediterranean Sauce	Chicken Breast in Spring Sauce
Red Wine and Cheese Snack	Cracker Pizza	Strawberry Cottage Cheese Snack	Glass of 2% Milk

Day 1

Breakfast: Ham Omelet with Fruit

Yield: 2 servings

Total time: 10 minutes

Ingredients:

8 egg whites

3 ounces lean ham, chopped

Salt and pepper to taste

Olive oil cooking spray

1 teaspoon extra-virgin olive oil

4 Wasa fiber crackers

Optional:

6 almonds

½ apple

½ orange

Whisk egg whites, ham, salt, and pepper together in a bowl. Lightly coat a skillet with cooking spray containing olive oil and set over medium heat. Add the egg mixture and tilt the skillet. As the egg mixture starts to cook, gently lift it with a spatula and continue to tilt the skillet so the uncooked egg mixture flows underneath to cook. Serve the omelet on crackers, or have the crackers on the side.

As an accompaniment, each omelet should have ½ apple, ½ orange, and 6 whole almonds as a side dish.

Per serving: Calories 341, protein 27 g, fat 11 g, carbohydrate 35 g, and
  fiber 8 g

Lunch: Balsamic Pork Fillet over Red Onions

Yield: 2 servings
Total time: 30 minutes

Ingredients:

Olive oil cooking spray

8 ounces pork fillet, cut into 2 pieces

4 small red onions, thinly sliced

3 teaspoons extra-virgin olive oil,
  divided

Salt and pepper to taste

2 tablespoons balsamic vinegar

1 apple, chopped

Spray a skillet with cooking spray and place over medium heat. Sauté the pork fillets for 5 minutes per side. Set aside.

In a stir-fry pan with 2 teaspoons of olive oil, stir-fry the thinly sliced onions. Season with salt and pepper and cook to desired consistency. Add the balsamic vinegar.

To serve, plate the hot onions. Top with the pork fillet cut into slices. Drizzle with the 1 teaspoon of remaining olive oil and garnish with the chopped apple.

Per serving: Calories 346, protein 28 g, fat 11 g, carbohydrate 34 g, and
  fiber 5 g

Late Afternoon Snack: Blueberry Ricotta Snack

Yield: 1 serving
Total time: 5 minutes

Ingredients:

⅓ cup blueberries   3 tablespoons low-fat ricotta

Stir the blueberries into the ricotta. (If you like it thinner, add a little water.)

Per serving: Calories 92, protein 6 g, fat 4 g, carbohydrate 10 g, and fiber 1 g

Dinner: Chicken Breast in Spring Sauce

Yield: 2 servings
Total time: 30 minutes

Ingredients:

6 ounces boneless, skinless chicken
    breast
Salt and pepper to taste
15 to 20 asparagus spears (about 1
    pound)
1 pound eggplant

½ cup unsalted vegetable stock
3 tablespoons plain low-fat yogurt
2 tablespoons chopped fresh chives
1 tablespoon extra-virgin olive oil
1 cup blueberries

Preheat the oven to 350°F. Season the chicken breast with salt and pepper and bake for 15 to 20 minutes. While the chicken is baking, peel and remove the woody parts of the asparagus ends; then chop the spears into 1-inch lengths. Peel the eggplant and cut into ½-inch cubes.

In a saucepan, bring the vegetable stock to a boil, reduce the heat, then add the diced eggplant and chopped asparagus, and cook for 7 minutes. Drain the vegetables, then mash them with the yogurt, chives, salt, and pepper.

Slice the chicken and divide the slices in half.

To serve, divide the vegetables over 2 plates, then top with the chicken slices. Drizzle the extra-virgin olive oil over the chicken and vegetables.

Enjoy 1 cup of blueberries per serving for dessert.

Per serving: Calories 357, protein 27 g, fat 10 g, carbohydrate 45 g, and
    fiber 16 g

Late-Night Snack: Deviled Eggs with Hummus

Yield: 2 servings (3 egg-white halves)
Total time: 2 minutes

Ingredients:

3 large hard-boiled eggs
6 tablespoons hummus

1½ teaspoons extra-virgin olive oil
Paprika for sprinkling

Slice the hard-boiled eggs in half, discarding the yolks. Fill each egg-white half with 1 tablespoon of hummus. Sprinkle all the egg-white halves with paprika.

Per serving: Calories 93, protein 8 g, fat 3 g, carbohydrate 8 g, and fiber 1 g

Total for Day 1: Calories 1,229, protein 96 g, fat 39 g, carbohydrate 132 g, and fiber 31 g

Day 2

Breakfast: Vegetable Omelet with Peanut Butter Crackers

Yield: 2 servings
Total time: 15 minutes

Ingredients:

10 large egg whites
Salt and pepper to taste
Olive oil cooking spray
1 teaspoon extra-virgin olive oil
1 medium tomato, chopped
2 cups fresh spinach, chopped

¼ cup shredded part-skim mozzarella
cheese
2 tablespoons reduced-fat peanut
butter
3 Wasa fiber crackers
1½ cups berries

Whisk egg whites, salt, and pepper together in a bowl. Set aside. Spray a skillet with cooking spray, add the olive oil, and place over medium heat. Cook the tomato and spinach for 1 minute, until the spinach wilts. Add the egg mixture, tilt skillet. As the egg mixture starts to cook, gently lift with a spatula and tilt skillet so the uncooked egg mixture flows underneath to cook. Add the cheese and cover for a minute or so to let the cheese melt some. Fold omelet in half and serve with peanut butter on Wasa and berries as a side dish.

Per serving: Calories 358, protein 30 g, fat 12 g, carbohydrate 37 g, and
fiber 9 g

Lunch: Beef and Broccoli

Yield: 2 servings
Total time: 20 minutes

Ingredients:

1 6-ounce lean top round steak	2 teaspoons lemon zest
1¼ pounds broccoli florets	Pinch ground cinnamon
½ cup unsalted vegetable stock	2 teaspoons extra-virgin olive oil
Salt and pepper to taste	1 small pear

Season the steak with salt and pepper and grill to your desired doneness. Set aside.

Bring a large pan of salted water to a boil. Add the broccoli, cook for about 7 minutes, and drain. In the cup of a blender, combine half of the florets with the vegetable stock and purée to get the right creamy consistency. Add salt and pepper. Combine the creamed broccoli to the broccoli florets in the pan.

To serve, divide the broccoli into 2 dishes. Sprinkle each with the lemon zest, cinnamon, and extra-virgin olive oil. Top with the steak cut into thin strips.

Enjoy a small pear for dessert.

Per serving: Calories 364, protein 27 g, fat 12 g, carbohydrate 46 g, and
fiber 12 g

Late Afternoon Snack: Bell Pepper and Hummus Snack

Yield: 1 serving
Total time: 5 minutes

Ingredients:

1 bell pepper, cut into strips
2 tablespoons hummus

3 grams whey protein powder

Mix whey protein into hummus in a small bowl. Spread hummus over bell pepper strips.

Per serving: Calories 91, protein 6 g, fat 3 g, carbohydrate 10 g, and fiber 4 g

Dinner: Grilled Sea Bass with Garlic Artichokes

Yield: 2 servings
Total time: 20 minutes

Ingredients:

6 teaspoons extra-virgin olive oil, divided
2 cloves garlic, sliced
14 ounces canned artichoke hearts, drained and quartered

Salt and pepper to taste
⅓ cup white wine
2 4-ounce sea bass fillets, cleaned and bones removed
1 teaspoon dried marjoram

Heat 2 teaspoons of the olive oil in a skillet over medium-low heat. Add the garlic to the skillet and let it flavor the oil. Remove the garlic. Add the artichoke hearts, salt, and pepper. Deglaze with the wine and cook for about 7 minutes. Set aside.

Coat a grill or grill pan with 2 teaspoons of the olive oil. Season the sea bass fillets with salt and marjoram, then grill 4 minutes per side.

Plate the artichokes and top with the sea bass fillets. Drizzle with the remaining extra virgin olive oil and serve.

Share a grapefruit as dessert.

Per serving: Calories 399, protein 28 g, fat 11 g, carbohydrate 46 g, and fiber 20 g

Late Night Snack: Quick Applesauce Snack

Yield: 1 serving

Total time: <5 minutes

Ingredients:

¼ cup unsweetened applesauce

¼ cup low-fat cottage cheese

½ teaspoon ground cinnamon
  (optional)

1½ teaspoons toasted slivered
  almonds

Combine the applesauce, cottage cheese, and cinnamon, if desired, in a bowl. Sprinkle the slivered almonds on top.

Per serving: Calories 91, protein 7 g, fat 3 g, carbohydrate 10 g, and fiber 1 g

Total for Day 2: Calories 1,303, protein 98 g, fat 41 g, carbohydrate 149 g, and fiber 46 g

Day 3

Breakfast: Yogurt and Berries

Yield: 2 servings

Total time: 5 minutes

Ingredients:

2 cups nonfat Greek yogurt

2 cups berries

½ cup slivered almonds

Stir all the ingredients together and serve in separate bowls.

Per serving: Calories 354, protein 30 g, fat 12 g, carbohydrate 36 g, and fiber 6 g

Lunch: Brussels Sprouts with Warm Goat Cheese

Yield: 2 servings

Total time: 25 minutes

Ingredients:

1¾ pounds Brussels sprouts, quartered

Salt to taste

Pepper to taste

3 ounces soft goat cheese

6 black olives, pitted and halved

2 tablespoons chopped fresh chives

1 kiwi fruit

Preheat the oven to 375°F. Add the Brussels sprouts to boiling salted water and cook for 10 to 15 minutes. While the Brussels sprouts are cooking, bake the goat cheese for 3 to 5 minutes, until it is warmed through and just starting to melt.

Drain the Brussels sprouts and combine with the warm goat cheese, salt, and pepper. Sprinkle with the olives and chives and serve in separate bowls.

Share a kiwi for dessert.

Per serving: Calories 343, protein 22 g, fat 12 g, carbohydrate 48 g, fiber 18 g

Late Afternoon Snack: Ham and Apple Snack

Yield: 2 servings

Total time: <5 minutes

Ingredients:

3 ounces (¼ pound) lean deli ham slices

1 small apple, cored and sliced

Wrap apple slices in each ham slice. Divide slices among 2 separate plates.

Per serving: Calories 100, protein 8 g, fat 4 g, carbohydrate 9 g, and fiber 1 g

Dinner: Lamb with Eggplant and Leek Salad

Yield: 2 servings

Total time: 30 minutes

Ingredients:

1 eggplant (about 1 pound)

Olive oil cooking spray

2 teaspoons extra-virgin olive oil, divided

⅔ pound leeks, thinly sliced

Salt to taste

2 tablespoons unsalted vegetable stock

8 ounces lean lamb loin

Pinch dried thyme

Pinch dried marjoram

Chili powder to taste

1 cup blueberries

Peel and pierce the eggplant a few times. Wrap in a wet paper towel, then cover with plastic wrap. Cook for 8 minutes in the microwave on high heat. While the eggplant cooks, coat the bottom of a skillet with olive oil spray and 1 teaspoon of the olive oil and place over medium heat. Sauté the leeks with salt for 10 minutes, adding stock as needed. Spray a second skillet with olive oil spray. Season the lamb loin with salt, thyme, and marjoram, and cook over medium heat, 6 minutes per side.

Cut the cooled eggplant into cubes and add to the sautéed leeks, and season with chili powder.

Put the eggplant and leek salad in a serving dish. Cut the lamb into slices and place on top of the eggplant and leek salad. Drizzle with the remaining 1 teaspoon extra-virgin olive oil and serve.

Serve ½ cup of blueberries per serving for dessert.

Per serving: Calories 364 g, protein 28 g, fat 11 g, carbohydrate 40 g, and fiber 12 g

Late Evening Snack: Turkey-Apple Crunch for Two

Yield: 2 servings
Total time: 10 minutes

Ingredients:

2 ounces cooked turkey, cubed
1 medium apple, cored and cubed

8 whole almonds

Divide the turkey and apple evenly with a friend, with the almonds on the side.

Per serving: Calories 97, protein 7 g, fat 3 g, carbohydrate 11 g, and fiber 2 g

Total for Day 3: Calories 1,258, protein 95 g, fat 42 g, carbohydrate 144 g, and fiber 39 g

Day 4

Breakfast: Salty Mousse

Yield: 2 servings
Total time: 5 minutes

Ingredients:

5 ounces fat-free cream cheese
4 ounces lean ham, chopped
15 olives, pitted and chopped

1¾ cups mixed berries
3 Wasa fiber crackers

Per serving: Calories 335, protein 25 g, fat 10 g, carbohydrate 38 g, and fiber 8 g

Lunch: Roasted Vegetables with Melted Mozzarella

Yield: 2 servings

Total time: 50 minutes

Ingredients:

Olive oil cooking spray

1 medium eggplant (about 1 pound)

3 medium tomatoes

1 bunch Belgian endive (about 1 pound)

1 small zucchini (about half a pound)

Salt and pepper to taste

9 large egg whites

2 tablespoons chopped chives

⅓ cup shredded part-skim mozzarella cheese

1 tablespoon extra-virgin olive oil

2 cups strawberries

Preheat the oven 425°F. Coat 2 baking sheets with cooking spray.

Slice the eggplant in half lengthwise, then cut each half into quarters lengthwise. Cut each in half crosswise to make two shorter quarters. Place the eggplant, skin side down, onto a prepared baking sheet. Cut the tomatoes and Belgian endive into halves. Cut the zucchini into ¾- to 1-inch-thick slices.

On the first baking sheet, arrange the eggplant and tomatoes and sprinkle with salt, pepper, and whatever spices you like. On the other baking sheet, arrange the endive and zucchini and sprinkle with salt, pepper, and whatever spices you like.

While the vegetables are roasting, mix the egg whites in a bowl. Add the chives, salt, and pepper. Set aside.

After 10 minutes, turn the endive. After 20 minutes, remove the endive from the baking sheet and turn the zucchini slices. After 25 to 30 minutes, remove the baking sheet containing the eggplant and tomatoes. After 40 minutes, remove the baking sheet containing the zucchini slices.

While the vegetables cool slightly, cook the egg white mixture in an olive oil–sprayed skillet.

Serve the vegetables on a plate, topped with the seasoned egg whites. Sprinkle with the mozzarella and return to the oven until mozzarella is melted. Drizzle with the extra virgin olive oil and serve.

Enjoy 1 cup strawberries per serving for dessert.

Per serving: Calories 386, protein 30 g, fat 12 g, carbohydrate 49 g, and fiber 22 g

Late Afternoon Snack: Pear and Parmesan Cheese Snack

Yield: 2 servings
Total time: 5 minutes

Ingredients:

3 ounces grated Parmesan   1 pear, cored and sliced

Top the pear slices with the grated cheese.

Per serving: Calories 103, protein 5 g, fat 4 g, carbohydrate 13 g, and fiber 3 g

Dinner: Chicken with Mushrooms and Peppers

Yield: 2 servings
Total time: 40 minutes

Ingredients:

3 teaspoons extra-virgin olive oil, divided

2 cloves garlic

3 red bell peppers, cored, seeded, and sliced

8 ounces sliced button mushrooms

1 medium onion, sliced

3 tablespoons unsalted vegetable stock

Salt and pepper to taste

7 ounces boneless, skinless chicken breast, sliced thin

10 ounces fresh spinach

2 tablespoons chopped fresh basil

1 cup cherries

Heat 1½ teaspoons of the extra-virgin olive oil in a skillet over medium heat. Add the garlic and cook until the cloves give off their aroma. Remove the garlic. Add the peppers to the skillet and cook for 2 minutes. Add the sliced mushrooms and onions, vegetable stock, salt, and pepper and cook for 6 minutes.

Add the chicken breast slices, cooking for about 5 minutes total and turning midway through cooking. Add the spinach and cook until wilted, about 2 minutes.

Turn the chicken mixture onto a serving plate. Garnish with the fresh basil, and drizzle the remaining 1½ teaspoons extra-virgin olive oil over the top.

Enjoy ½ cup cherries per serving for dessert.

Per serving: Calories 360, protein 32 g, fat 11 g, carbohydrate 38 g, and fiber 11 g

Late Night Snack: Red Wine and Cheese Snack

Yield: 1 serving

Total time: <5 minutes

Ingredients:

4 ounces red wine   1 stick light string cheese

Per serving: Calories 142, protein 7 g, fat 3 g, carbohydrate 3 g, fiber 0 g

Total for Day 4: Calories 1,326, protein 99 g, fat 40 g, carbohydrate 141 g, and fiber 44 g

Day 5

Breakfast: Spinach Omelet with Fruit Bowl

Yield: 2 servings

Total time: 20 minutes

Ingredients:

1 pear, cored and chopped

2 kiwi fruits, peeled and chopped

Juice of 1 lemon

8 whole almonds, chopped

10 large egg whites

Black pepper to taste

Olive oil cooking spray

1 teaspoon extra-virgin olive oil

2 cups spinach, chopped

¼ cup grated Parmesan cheese

3 Wasa fiber crackers

Drizzle the pear and kiwi with the lemon juice and toss. Place in two bowls and top with the almonds.

Whisk the egg whites and pepper together in a bowl. Coat the bottom of a skillet with olive oil spray and the extra-virgin olive oil, heat to medium, and cook the spinach for 1 minute, or until wilted. Add the egg mixture and tilt the skillet. As the egg mixture starts to cook, gently lift with a spatula and tilt the skillet so the uncooked egg mixture flows underneath to cook. Add the Parmesan and cover for 1 minute. Fold the cooked egg mixture in half and serve with the crackers and a fruit bowl.

Per serving: Calories 345, protein 28 g, fat 10 g, carbohydrate 39 g, and
fiber 10 g

Lunch: Orange Grilled Salmon with Fennel Tomato Salad

Yield: 2 servings
Total time: 20 minutes

Ingredients:

¼ cup freshly squeezed orange juice

1½ teaspoons extra-virgin olive oil

Salt and pepper to taste

2 3½-ounce salmon fillets

Pinch paprika

2 pounds fennel, thinly sliced

3 medium tomatoes, diced

1 cup raspberries

In a medium bowl, combine the orange juice, extra-virgin olive oil, salt, and pepper and emulsify. Pour two tablespoons of the orange juice mixture over the salmon, sprinkle with the paprika, and let sit 10 minutes.

In a medium bowl, combine the fennel and tomatoes and season with the remaining orange oil emulsion.

Over medium-high heat, grill the salmon in a pan on the stove for 4 minutes per side.

Plate the salmon alongside the vegetables.

Enjoy a small bowl of raspberries for dessert.

Per serving: Calories 399, protein 29 g, fat 12 g, carbohydrate 50 g, and
fiber 22 g

Late Afternoon Snack: Berries and Yogurt

Yield: 1 serving

Total time: 5 minutes

Ingredients:

¼ cup nonfat Greek yogurt

¼ cup berries

4 whole almonds

Mix the yogurt and berries together in a bowl. Have the nuts on the side for crunch or chop them and blend into the yogurt.

Per serving: Calories 82, protein 7 g, fat 3 g, carbohydrate 9 g, and fiber 1 g

Dinner: Turkey with Sautéed Zucchini

Yield: 2 servings

Total time: 30 minutes

Ingredients:

Olive oil cooking spray

3 teaspoons extra-virgin olive oil, divided

2 pounds cubed zucchini

2 small onions, diced

2 tablespoons unsalted vegetable stock

6 ounces cubed turkey breast

Salt and pepper to taste

¼ cup chopped fresh parsley

12 black olives, sliced

1 cup pineapple

Coat the bottom of a skillet with olive oil spray, then add 1 teaspoon of the olive oil and place the skillet over high heat. Add the zucchini and onions and cook for about 6 minutes, adding stock as needed. Add the cubed turkey breast, salt, and pepper and cook for another 5 minutes.

To serve, plate the turkey and vegetables, then garnish with the parsley and sliced olives. Drizzle with the remaining 2 teaspoons extra-virgin olive oil.

Enjoy ½ cup pineapple per serving for dessert.

Per serving: Calories 343, protein 28 g, fat 11 g, carbohydrate 38 g, and fiber 9 g

Late Night Snack: Cracker Pizza

Yield: 1 serving
Total time: 10 minutes

Ingredients:

1½ Wasa fiber crackers
2 tablespoons part-skim mozzarella
cheese, shredded

3 tablespoons tomato salsa

Preheat the oven to 450°F.

Place the crackers on a small baking sheet. Divide the mozzarella equally atop the crackers. Bake for about 5 minutes, or until the cheese has melted.

Serve with the salsa.

Per serving: Calories 108, protein 6 g, fat 3 g, carbohydrate 14 g, and fiber 4 g

Total for Day 5: Calories 1,277, protein 98 g, fat 39 g, carbohydrate 150 g, and fiber 46 g

Day 6

Breakfast: Fruit Mousse

Yield: 2 servings
Total time: 15 minutes

Ingredients:

7 ounces low-fat ricotta (about
1 cup)
2 tablespoons sugar-free preserves,
any flavor
12 whole almonds, sliced

3½ teaspoons whey protein powder
1 cup 2% milk
3 Wasa fiber crackers
1 apple, cored and sliced

Blend the ricotta, preserves, and almonds in a blender until smooth. Stir the Zone protein powder into the milk. Combine with the ricotta mixture.

To serve, spread a layer of mousse on the crackers, then top with the apple slices.

Per serving: Calories 327, protein 25 g, fat 11 g, carbohydrate 40 g, and
fiber 11 g

Lunch: Shrimp Salad with Green Beans, Hearts of Palm, and Tomatoes

Yield: 2 servings
Total time: 50 minutes

Ingredients:

½ pound large unpeeled (31/35) shrimp, deveined

1 bay leaf

1 pound green beans, chopped in 1-inch lengths

⅓ cup chopped hearts of palm

2 small tomatoes, chopped

2 tablespoons freshly squeezed lemon juice

4 teaspoons extra-virgin olive oil

2 teaspoons ground thyme

Salt and pepper to taste

1 cup strawberries

Drop the raw shrimp into boiling water along with the bay leaf and cook for 1 to 2 minutes. Remove the pot from the heat, cover, and allow the shrimp to continue cooking in the hot water for 5 to 10 minutes, depending on the size of the shrimp. (They should be pink and opaque.) Pour the shrimp into a strainer to drain them, removing the bay leaf. When the shrimp are cool to the touch, peel and cut into bite-sized pieces.

While the shrimp are cooking, in a separate pot, cook the cut green beans for about 5 minutes, or until tender-crisp. Time the beans to be done at the same time as the shrimp.

In a medium bowl, combine the hearts of palm and tomatoes, then season with the lemon juice, extra-virgin olive oil, thyme, salt, and pepper. Add the shrimp and green beans and combine. Serve at room temperature.

Enjoy ½ cup strawberries per serving for dessert.

Per serving: Calories 368, protein 30 g, fat 12 g, carbohydrate 40 g, and
fiber 10 g

Late Afternoon Snack: Chocolate Mousse Snack

Yield: 1 serving
Total time: 5 minutes

Ingredients:

⅓ ounce unsweetened baker's chocolate, melted (about ¼ square)

½ cup plain fat-free yogurt
3 whole almonds, chopped

In a microwave-safe bowl, melt the chocolate in the microwave, at low heat, for 10 to 20 seconds, or longer if needed. (Work in 10-second increments to avoid overheating the chocolate.)

Blend the chocolate with the yogurt to obtain a mousse-like consistency. Add the almonds and stir to combine.

Per serving: Calories 107, protein 7 g, fat 3 g, carbohydrate 13 g, and fiber 3 g

Dinner: Veal in Mediterranean Sauce

Yield: 2 servings
Total time: 45 minutes

Ingredients:

1 medium spaghetti squash
7 ounces veal, filleted and sliced
3½ teaspoons extra-virgin olive oil, divided
Pinch fresh thyme leaves
Pinch ground marjoram
1 clove garlic
3 tablespoons chopped fresh basil

2 tablespoons unsalted vegetable stock (or more as needed)
3 pounds tomatoes, peeled and diced
Salt and pepper to taste
1 teaspoon dried oregano
1 tablespoon chopped fresh parsley
1 medium apricot

Carefully pierce the squash six or seven times with a fork. In a microwave-safe bowl, cook the spaghetti squash in the microwave on high for 10 to12 minutes, turning halfway. Cook until a fork inserts easily through the skin and into the flesh of the squash. Repeat in 2-minute increments until you can insert the fork. Let stand at least 5 minutes. (The squash will be HOT.) Holding the squash with a towel or gloves, cut it in half lengthwise. Scoop out the seeds and fibers with a large spoon and discard. Use a fork to separate the strands and scrape the flesh out of the shell. Set aside.

Marinate the sliced veal fillet for at least 10 minutes in a mixture prepared with the extra-virgin olive oil, thyme, and marjoram.

Make the Mediterranean sauce: In a skillet over medium heat, sauté the garlic and basil for 1 minute with the vegetable stock. Add the diced tomatoes and cook for 15 minutes.

While the Mediterranean sauce is cooking, preheat a skillet and sauté the veal slices 1 minute per side, or until lightly browned. Add the Mediterranean sauce to the veal and cook for 2 minutes. Season with the salt, pepper, and oregano. Sprinkle with the chopped parsley and serve over the spaghetti squash.

Share an apricot for dessert.

Per serving: Calories 351, protein 27 g, fat 12 g, carbohydrate 40 g, and fiber 11 g

Late Evening Snack: Strawberry Cottage Cheese Snack

Yield: 1 serving
Total time: 5 minutes

Ingredients:

¾ cup strawberries   3 almonds
¼ cup low-fat cottage cheese

Add sliced strawberries to cottage cheese in a bowl. Sprinkle with the almonds.

Per serving: Calories 104, protein 8 g, fat 3 g, carbohydrate 11 g, and fiber 3 g

Total for Day 6: Calories 1,257, protein 97 g, fat 41 g, carbohydrate 134 g, and fiber 28 g

Breakfast: Ham and Strawberry Cream Cheese Crackers

Yield: 2 servings

Total time: 10 minutes

Ingredients:

6 ounces fat-free cream cheese

4 macadamia nuts, chopped small

4 ounces lean ham, chopped

1 pint strawberries, divided

4 Wasa fiber crackers

In a medium bowl, mix the cream cheese with the chopped macadamia nuts, ham, and ⅓ of the strawberries. Spread the mixture on the crackers and have the rest of the strawberries on the side.

Per serving: Calories 367, protein 28 g, fat 12 g, carbohydrate 39 g, and fiber 10 g

Lunch: Orange-Vanilla Halibut with Onions and Artichoke Hearts

Yield: 2 servings

Total time: 20 minutes

Ingredients:

2 medium sweet onions, coarsely chopped

14 ounces canned artichoke hearts, rinsed and drained

1 vanilla bean, cut lengthwise

½ cup unsalted vegetable stock

2 3½-ounce halibut fillets

Zest of 2 oranges

4 teaspoons extra-virgin olive oil

Salt and pepper to taste

2 oranges

In a skillet over medium heat, combine the onions and artichoke hearts with the vanilla bean and vegetable stock, and cook just until onions start to soften. Remove the vanilla bean.

Steam the fish with the zest of 1 orange for about 8 minutes.

Plate the artichoke heart/onion mixture. Top each plate with the fish. Drizzle with the extra-virgin olive oil, and sprinkle with salt and pepper.

Enjoy an orange per serving for dessert.

Per serving: Calories 399, protein 29 g, fat 12 g, carbohydrate 50 g, and fiber 22 g

Late Afternoon Snack: Whey Blueberry Snack

Yield: 1 serving
Total time: 5 minutes

Ingredients:

1½ teaspoons whey protein powder	½ cup blueberries
8 ounces water	4 whole almonds

Stir the whey protein powder into the water. Blend with the berries in a blender. Have the almonds on the side for crunch.

Per serving: Calories 97, protein 7 g, fat 3 g, carbohydrate 13 g, and fiber 3 g

Dinner: Chicken Breast in Spring Sauce

Yield: 2 servings
Total time: 30 minutes

Ingredients:

6 ounces boneless, skinless chicken breast	½ cup unsalted vegetable stock
Salt and pepper to taste	3 tablespoons plain low-fat yogurt
15 to 20 asparagus spears (about 1 pound)	2 tablespoons chopped fresh chives
1 eggplant (about 1 pound)	1 tablespoon extra-virgin olive oil
	1 cup blueberries

Preheat the oven to 350°F. Season the chicken breast with salt and pepper and bake for 15 to 20 minutes. While the chicken is baking, peel and remove the woody parts of the asparagus ends; then chop the spears into 1-inch lengths. Peel the eggplant and cut into ½-inch cubes.

In a saucepan, bring the vegetable stock to a boil, reduce the heat, then add the diced eggplant and chopped asparagus, and cook for 7 minutes. Drain the vegetables, then mash them with the yogurt, chives, salt, and pepper.

Slice the chicken and divide the slices in half.

To serve, divide the vegetables over 2 plates, then top with the chicken slices. Drizzle the extra-virgin olive oil over the chicken and vegetables.

Enjoy 1 cup of blueberries per serving for dessert.

Per serving: Calories 357, protein 27 g, fat 10 g, carbohydrate 45 g, and fiber 16 g

Late Night Snack: Glass of 2% Milk

Yield: 1 serving
Total time: <1 minute

Ingredients:

6 ounces 2% milk

Pour and enjoy!

Per serving: Calories 98, protein 6 g, fat 4 g, carbohydrate 8 g, and fiber 0 g

Total for Day 7: Calories 1,318, protein 97 g, fat 41 g, carbohydrate 155 g, and fiber 51 g

Shopping List for a Week in the Mediterranean Zone

LEAN MEATS AND FISH
- chicken breast, boneless, skinless
- eggs, egg whites
- halibut
- ham (lean)
- lamb loin (lean)
- pork (lean)
- top round steak (lean)
- salmon
- sea bass
- shrimp
- turkey
- veal

VEGETABLES
- artichoke hearts
- asparagus
- bell peppers
- black olives
- broccoli
- Brussels sprouts
- chives
- eggplant
- fennel
- garlic
- green beans
- hearts of palm
- leeks
- mushrooms
- onions, red
- spaghetti squash
- spinach
- tomatoes
- zucchini

FRUIT
- apples
- applesauce, unsweetened
- apricots
- blackberries
- blueberries
- cherries
- grapefruit
- kiwis
- lemons
- oranges
- pears
- pineapple
- raspberries
- strawberries

DAIRY
- cream cheese, fat-free
- Greek yogurt, fat-free
- goat cheese
- cottage cheese, low-fat
- milk, 2%
- mozzarella cheese, part-skim
- Parmesan
- ricotta, part-skim
- string (mozzarella) cheese, light
- yogurt, plain, low-fat

PANTRY & REFRIGERATOR STAPLES
- almonds
- basil, fresh
- bay leaf, dried
- chili powder
- cinnamon, ground

hummus	salsa
olive oil	salt
olive oil cooking spray	thyme, ground
macadamia nuts	chocolate, unsweetened baker's
marjoram	vanilla bean
paprika	vegetable stock, low-sodium
parsley	Wasa fiber crackers
peanut butter, reduced-fat	whey protein
peppers, bell	wine, red and white
preserves, sugar-free	

Each of these seven days in the Mediterranean Zone illustrates the Zone Paradox. You are eating a lot of food but not a lot of calories. None of the meals supplies more than 400 calories and every day in the Mediterranean Zone provides less than 1,400 calories, yet you are neither hungry nor fatigued since you are stabilizing blood sugar levels. The maximum protein in any day in the Mediterranean Zone is only slightly less than what average Americans are currently eating, and the fiber content is dramatically greater than the typical American diet. I should also add the total fat content in the Mediterranean Zone never exceeds 50 grams per day, which is considered a low-fat diet. Frankly, who could argue with a diet like that for a lifetime?

A week in the Mediterranean Zone is really only a glimpse into a lifetime in the Mediterranean Zone. You can change meals very simply by making different protein substitutions. For vegetarians, simply take out three ounces of chicken or beef and replace it with three ounces of low-fat cheese, six egg whites, six ounces of extra-firm tofu, or three ounces of a soy imitation-meat product (the last two protein sources are for vegans). Alternatively, you can replace the three ounces of low-fat protein with four and a half ounces of fish or six ounces of a low-fat dairy product. It doesn't take much effort to quickly make a large cookbook of Mediterranean Zone meals that can fit into any dietary philosophy.

What if you are losing too much fat and you can actually begin to see your abdominal muscles? Then simply take out the late afternoon snack and replace it with another Mediterranean Zone meal or add a handful of nuts to your late afternoon or evening snack.

What if you wanted to the take the Mediterranean Zone to its most extreme, using only Paleolithic ingredients? Would you get better results? Probably. The only problem with the Mediterranean PaleoZone is potential dietary boredom due to the decreased number of food ingredients you can use: no alcohol, no dairy products (milk or cheese), no legumes, and no grains. This rather draconian approach to the Mediterranean Zone is also difficult to adhere to (the lack of alcohol is usually the primary complaint) for an extended period of time.

Even if you follow a Paleolithic version of the Mediterranean Zone, you still need to supplement your diet with additional omega-3 fatty acids and polyphenols to reduce cellular inflammation to its lowest levels and simultaneously reach the clinical markers that define the Zone. Of course, adding anti-inflammatory supplements also lets you live a little more on the dietary wild side so that you can enjoy an occasional glass of red wine, a cup of cappuccino, or some traditional dark chocolate that contains a little sugar and milk to reduce the bitterness of its high polyphenol content.

How anti-inflammatory supplements work to enhance the foundation of the Mediterranean Zone is discussed in the next chapter.

6

Anti-inflammatory Supplements for the Mediterranean Zone

The Mediterranean Zone can be defined as a lifetime eating plan that helps your body maintain your inflammatory response within a healthy range. What makes the Mediterranean diet useful in managing inflammatory responses are ample polyphenols from fruits and vegetables and omega-3 fatty acids from fish coupled with decreased intake of omega-6 and saturated fatty acids.

The Mediterranean Zone enhances the anti-inflammatory control of the Mediterranean diet by giving it more structure, especially in the balance of protein to the glycemic load, to enhance its hormonal responses. But to get the full anti-inflammatory benefits of the Mediterranean Zone you will still probably have to consider supplementing it with additional purified omega-3 fatty acids and purified extracts rich in polyphenols.

PURIFIED OMEGA-3 FATTY ACIDS

Until recently, eating a lot of fish was a relatively easy approach to getting adequate levels of omega-3 fatty acids in the diet. Fish was cheap, and it was safe to eat. Those days are over. Because of technological advances, we are hunting fish into extinction, and as a result, the cost of fish is skyrocketing. Second, we have been using the oceans as a dumping ground for toxic chemicals that have been accumulating in the fish we eat. The end result of both factors is a decreasing consumption of fish, which means a decreasing intake of anti-inflammatory omega-3 fatty acids.

So just how much omega-3 fatty acids do you need if your goal is to keep yourself in the Zone? I believe you will need a minimum of 2.5 grams of omega-3 fatty acids per day. These are not just any omega-3 fatty acids, but the longer chain omega-3 fatty acids, eicosapentaenoic acid (EPA) and docosahexaenoic acid (DHA), found only in fish and fish oil concentrates. The average American consumes about 125 mg of EPA and DHA per day, or about 5 percent of my minimum recommended omega-3 fatty acid dose.

It wasn't always that way. At the turn of the twentieth century, fish consumption was high, and if your grandparents didn't eat a lot of fish, then your great-grandparents would have given them a daily tablespoon of cod liver oil. While cod liver oil was the most disgusting food known to man (perhaps the only exception would be garum—see previous chapter!), a daily tablespoon of cod liver oil did provide 2.5 grams of EPA and DHA. Unfortunately, cod liver oil today is heavily contaminated with toxins, especially polychlorinated biphenyls (PCBs). Sadly, those toxic chemicals haven't improved the taste, either.

You could eat more fish to get the minimum levels of EPA and DHA for the Mediterranean Zone, but to get 2.5 grams of EPA and DHA per day, you'd have to eat:

- 6 pounds of lobster per day
- 2 pounds of tuna per day
- ⅓ pound of farmed salmon per day

Each of these solutions has some problems. Let's start with the lobster. It's expensive, and it also contains virtually no EPA and DHA. People like to eat it because it doesn't have a fishy taste, but unless you have both an unlimited budget and an unlimited taste for crustaceans, that's not going to work. Tuna is accessible and affordable, but is contaminated with mercury. In fact, the EPA recommends you eat no more than six ounces of albacore ("white") tuna or twelve ounces of canned light tuna per week.

Farm-raised salmon is lower in mercury but still high in PCBs. (Sidebar: 95 percent of all salmon consumed is farm-raised. Unfortunately, they are fed crude fish oil rich in PCBs so that the final product you get in a restaurant has five times the levels of PCBs compared to more expensive wild salmon.)

A far better way to ensure you get the necessary 2.5 grams of EPA and DHA per day that your grandparents got when they took their tablespoon of cod liver oil is to use highly purified omega-3 fatty acids that are also free of mercury and extremely low in PCBs.

This is trickier than it looks, because the fat-soluble toxins (PCBs, dioxins, and flame retardants, for example) in fish become concentrated in the crude fish oil when it is extracted. These compounds are known neurotoxins, carcinogens, and endocrine disruptors. This means they cause damage to the nervous system, increase the incidence of cancer, and cause hormonal disruptions, such as making you fat. Consider crude fish oil as the sewer of the sea—a collection vehicle for fat-soluble toxins. Once these toxins enter your body, they go directly to the organs in your body that contain the most fat and stay there. Those target organs are your brain and organs rich in fat cells (primarily your adipose tissue).

The solution to removing most of this contamination in fish oils was developed about fifteen years ago with the implementation of sophisticated new refining techniques that not only removed the majority of toxins, but also concentrated the omega-3 fatty acids. Unfortunately, most fish oil products available for the consumer don't use this sophisticated technology, so it remains "caveat emptor"—buyer beware—when it comes to omega-3 fatty acid supplements in the supermarket or local health food store. Given that precaution, what things should you look for in a fish oil supplement?

The first factors are color, smell, and taste. There are many wine connoisseurs (most seem to be located in California), but very few fish oil connoisseurs (I happen to be one). The best way to test a good wine is exactly the best way to test for good fish oil. Just as a wine should be clear to the eye, the same is true of refined fish oil. If the fish oil capsule is cloudy, you can be assured that the oil inside is probably contaminated with toxins such as PCBs.

So why are PCBs so bad for you? PCBs were used as an insulating fluid for electric transformers in the twentieth century. At the time they were considered inert chemicals. However, in 1979 PCB production was banned in the United States and eventually stopped worldwide in 2001 because of their toxicity. Unfortunately, by that time millions of pounds of PCBs had been dumped into lakes, rivers, and oceans. Since PCBs are virtually indestructible (that is why they were such a good insulator for electronic transformers), they accumulate through the marine food chain, eventually ending up concentrated in fish. When you eat the fish at the top of the food chain, you are also getting a lot of PCBs. The only way to measure PCBs is with incredibly expensive analytical equipment. So unless you have a half-million-dollar machine in your kitchen, then how do you know?

There is one simple test of fish oil purity that doesn't require a lot of sophisticated equipment. Simply break open four or five fish oil capsules and empty the contents into a shot glass. Put the shot glass in the freezer. Then come back five hours later with a toothpick. If you can't put the toothpick through the fish oil (meaning it is frozen solid), this is a good indication that your fish oil is probably the "sewer of the sea." If you can put a toothpick through it, it might be OK. I say *might be*, because it can still contain high levels of PCBs.

This is why you should never trust anyone in the fish oil industry to tell you the truth. When I wrote my book *The OmegaRx Zone*, which started the fish oil revolution more than a decade ago, I warned of this problem. Since then, many more people consume fish oils believing they are pure. So here are the four dirty secrets of fish oil marketing you should be aware of:

Dirty Secret #1. All fish oils contain PCBs.

The industrial chemicals (such as PCBs) that have been dumped into the rivers and oceans for the past two generations ensure that every fish in the world today is contaminated. Stating that any fish or fish oil is totally free from PCBs is simply a lie. Drug companies selling prescription fish oil products often make the statement that their fish oil is completely free of PCBs. Good marketing, but bad science. While prescription fish oil products are lower in PCBs than what you buy in a supermarket or health food store, they definitely are not free of these toxins.

Recently the state of California began to require warning labels on any food product (and that includes fish oils) that contains more than 90 nanograms of PCBs in a recommended daily dose. A nanogram (ng) is like a single drop of water in a large swimming pool. Because of the levels of PCBs in many popular consumer brands of fish oils, recommending more than a single capsule per day would force a manufacturer to have a warning label on its bottle stating it may be dangerous to your health. In fact, eight fish oil manufacturers were sued by environmentalists in 2010 because they were not disclosing the true value of PCBs in their products. They were reporting less than 4 percent of the 209 total PCB isomers in order to claim that their products met the new standards in California. The fish oil manufacturers lost the lawsuit, and now all fish oil products have to report the true levels of PCBs.

When *Consumer Reports*, a leading consumer magazine in the United States, investigated a number of fish oils in its January 2012 issue, its researchers found several national American brands were so high in PCBs that one or two capsules would have exceeded the maximum intake of total PCB levels set by the state of California. Before taking your next fish oil capsule, go to the website of the manufacturer and search for the technical data on the levels of all 209 isomers of PCBs in that particular lot of the company's product. If the product isn't there, then assume that the maximum amount of fish oil you should be consuming is about one gram (that's usually one capsule). Unfortunately, one fish oil capsule a day will not get you very close to my recommendations of 2.5 grams of EPA and DHA daily, but at least you are protecting yourself from PCBs accumulating in your fat cells and in your brain.

Dirty Secret #2. "Natural" fish oil is often unnatural.

Natural fish oil needs only to be heated to release the stored fats from the fish. Unfortunately, the maximum levels of omega-3 fatty acids in these natural fish oils is never greater than 30 percent of the total fatty acids. Natural fish oil, however, can then be refined to make much more concentrated omega-3 fatty acid products. The more refined the fish oil, the higher the levels of omega-3 fatty acids and the lower the levels of PCBs it will contain than in natural fish oils (especially cod liver oil). This is one case where refined is better than "natural."

Furthermore, other "fish oils" (such as krill oil) are not really fish oil. Krill are small shrimp that are dissolved in gasoline (hexane) and then treated with nail polish remover (acetone) to get the final product. This is also how you purify soy lecithin, an emulsifier used in many, many pre-packaged foods, from reduced-fat margarine to cooking sprays. (This is another little secret of the health food industry.) A substantial amount of the fatty acids in krill oil are actually free fatty acids, which are very prone to oxidation. So in addition to having low levels of omega-3 fatty acids compared to fish oil concentrates and high levels of easily oxidized free fatty acids, krill oil still contains PCBs.

To get rid of PCBs from any fish oil or krill oil, you first have to make ethyl esters from the extracted crude fish oil. This requires ethanol, which, unlike hexane or acetone, is not particularly harmful to you (since ethanol is the alcohol in wine). From these ethyl esters you can then distill out the vast majority of the remaining PCBs, making it safe to consume (see Dirty Secret #1). The vast majority of human clinical studies with omega-3 fatty acids have been done with omega-3 fatty acid concentrates consisting of purified ethyl esters low in PCBs.

However, you can process ethyl esters further to make a reconstituted "natural" triglyceride. Unfortunately, the postioning of the omega-3 fatty acids is now a totally different configuration than the true natural fish oil in the wild. As a result, these "natural" triglycerides are not natural at all.

Dirty Secret #3. Most fish oil can easily go rancid.

The freshness of any edible oil is determined by its rancidity. This is measured by its total oxidation (Totox) value. The World Health Organization (WHO) has set the upper Totox value at 26 milliequivalents per kilogram (mEq/kg). Any Totox number higher than 26 indicates the product is rancid. Many poorly refined fish oils have significant odor problems because of the presence of oxidation products consisting of aldehydes and ketones. As a result, marketers often add flavors to them and market them as "fresh." In reality, these flavors do nothing more than mask the smell of fish oil that still often exceeds Totox limits, making it unsuitable for human consumption as judged by World Health Organization standards. Because the omega-3 fatty acids are extremely prone to oxidation (even after they are put into a capsule or bottle), the only way to ensure that a fish oil product is not rancid is to test its Totox levels after it is has been bottled or encapsulated. A good quality fish oil company will post both the PCB and Totox levels of every batch of fish oil they sell on their website.

Dirty Secret #4. Fish oil won't help, unless you take enough.

The typical American diet is so low in omega-3 fatty acids and so rich in omega-6 fatty acids that you'd need a lot of purified fish oil to make a difference. Since omega-6 fatty acids are the cheapest form of calories known, they now represent the single largest item in the American diet. To get a better balance of omega-6 to omega-3 fatty acids, the average American is going to have to eat a lot of fish (such as the Japanese) or take a lot of purified omega-3 fatty acids as a supplement to have any significant reduction in cellular inflammation. This is why so many clinical studies with fish have conflicting results. They often give the subjects in the study too little omega-3 fatty acids to make a significant change in the balance of omega-3 to omega-6 fatty acids and thus the levels of cellular inflammation. If you give a placebo dose of omega-3 fatty acids, then you can expect placebo results.

The only way you can determine if you are eating enough fish or fish oil (both are highly unlikely) or consuming too many omega-6 fatty acids from vegetable oils (highly likely) is a blood test. In particular, you are looking for the level of the omega-6 fatty acid arachidonic acid (AA), the primary indicator of the level of pro-inflammatory responses in the body, relative to the level of the omega-3 fatty acid eicosapentaenoic acid (EPA), the primary indicator of the level of anti-inflammatory resolution responses in the body. You need a balance of both fatty acids to maintain a healthy inflammatory response. That balance can be found in your AA/EPA ratio in the blood. The lower the AA/EPA ratio is, the less cellular inflammation you have in your body. This is why I use this blood test as one of the key clinical markers of being in the Zone.

Ideally, you want to be taking in enough purified omega-3 fatty acids so that the AA/EPA ratio in the blood is between 1.5 and 3. (See the chart in Chapter 3.) The lower the AA/EPA ratio you have, the less cellular inflammation your body is exposed to. For comparison, the AA/EPA ratio is 1.5

in the Japanese, who are the longest-lived individuals in the world with the least amount of age-related disability (in other words, they age better). For Americans, the average AA/EPA ratio is about 20. For years, the Mediterranean population was somewhat between these two ranges. However, a recent study in Italy indicated that the older population still has a relatively low AA/EPA ratio (about 10), but the younger population now has an AA/EPA ratio similar to Americans (about 20). Our twin epidemics of obesity and diabetes are direct consequences of the growing imbalance of AA and EPA in our bodies, which has led to increased cellular inflammation. As you can see from the changes in the AA/EPA ratio in the Italian population (especially the younger generation), our cellular inflammation problem is spreading to the Mediterranean region. This may explain why, in one generation, Italian children have gone from being the leanest in Europe to among the fattest.

How much purified, omega-3-rich fish oil you have to take to control cellular inflammation depends on how closely you are following the Mediterranean Zone. The more you control diet-induced inflammation by following the Mediterranean Zone, then the less purified omega-3 fatty acids you will need to reduce cellular inflammation. On the other hand, the more white carbohydrates (bread, pasta, rice, and potatoes) you eat and the more omega-6 fatty acids (coming from vegetable oils) you consume, the more purified omega-3 fatty acids you will also need to consume to restore the necessary AA/EPA ratio into a range consistent for a healthy, balanced inflammatory response in your body.

My book *The OmegaRx Zone* was subtitled *The Miracle of High-Dose Fish Oil*. Let me give you three examples of the power of high levels of supplemental omega-3 fatty acids to support that subtitle.

EXAMPLE #1: Probably the most serious injury to the brain is severe brain trauma resulting in deep coma. The likelihood of emerging from that coma is usually slim to none. My first experience with such a patient occurred in 2006 after the Sago Mine (West Virginia) disaster, in which thirteen miners were trapped in a cave-in surrounded by high levels of carbon monoxide for forty-one hours. When the miners were finally rescued, only one, Randall McCloy, was still alive, but just barely. He was rushed to the nearest national brain trauma center, which was under the direction of Julian Bailes, one of the top neurosurgeons in the country. When Randall was examined at the trauma center, he had heart failure, kidney failure, liver failure, and brain failure. The brain failure came from being exposed to more than forty hours of high carbon monoxide levels that had destroyed much of the white matter in his brain. That night I got a call from Julian saying that since he had read my book *The OmegaRx Zone*, he thought that fish oil might help keep Randall McCloy from dying. I told him we should start with about 15 grams of EPA and DHA per day and his response was, "Oh my God, he will bleed to death." I assured Julian that Randall would not bleed to death because I would use continued testing to make sure that his AA/EPA ratio never fell below 1.5, which is the average in the Japanese population, and they certainly don't bleed to death. That night I air-shipped several bottles of highly purified liquid omega-3 fatty acids to Julian. He still had to fight the other members of the medical team on the use of that level of omega-3 fatty acids, but he convinced them that this was Randall's only hope.

Every day Randall was fed 15 grams of purified omega-3 fatty acids through his feeding tube. Of course, we were constantly measuring his AA/EPA ratio during that time, and it never went below 3. After two months on high-dose fish oil, he came out of his coma. The same dose was continued with oral feeding, using a tablespoon as a low-tech delivery system. Four months after the mine disaster, he was discharged to go home. His heart was normal, his kidney function was normal, his liver was normal, and he gave a speech to the media that would rival that of any politician. The press announced it a miracle, but in reality it was the aggressive use of high-dose omega-3 fatty acids to reduce the inflammation in his heart, liver, kidneys, and, of course, brain.

Was it a lucky break? Maybe not. Since that time, Julian Bailes has used the same protocol to help bring other patients back from the dead. Nonetheless, when I offer the same fish oil for free to medical schools for compassionate use in their severe brain trauma patients, I usually get a polite refusal because they fear the patients will bleed to death.

EXAMPLE #2: Severe brain trauma is one thing, but what about mild brain trauma such as that found in concussion injuries? A number of retired NFL players suffer greatly from past concussion injuries. I have had the opportunity to work with many of these ex-NFL athletes, but one of the most interesting is George Visger. George played for the San Francisco

49ers in the early 1980s. When I met him a few years ago, he had already had nine operations to relieve constant swelling in his brain caused by repeated football-related head traumas, and he essentially had no short-term memory. His day literally revolved around taking copious notes of everything he did that hour so he could refer back to his notebooks the next day to maintain a record of his life. I told George that based on cases with severe brain trauma patients, such as Randall McCloy, I knew that high-dose omega-3 fatty acids could help. Since his lack of short-term memory was also matched by his ADHD, I started him on the same levels of omega-3 fatty acids I used to treat children with ADHD as well as those with severe brain trauma (15 grams of EPA and DHA per day). Within a relatively short period of time, George's short-term memory significantly improved until one day he told me he actually remembered the previous day's events without writing them down. Today, George is an accomplished and passionate speaker as an advocate for more aggressive care for those living with the long-term consequences of concussion damage.

EXAMPLE #3: Another extension of the brain we often forget to consider is our sight. Most people's greatest fear of aging is dementia. Their second biggest fear is going blind. The primary cause of blindness as you age is a condition called age-related macular degeneration (AMD), the leading cause of blindness after age 50. There is no treatment for AMD. Once you get it, you will eventually go legally blind.

To determine the potential of high-dose fish oil to treat AMD, we used between 5 and 10 grams of omega-3 fatty acids. With AMD, the success of any therapy is easily evaluated by the patient's ability to read letters on an eye chart, similar to the one you use in getting your driver's license. If the improvement in vision was 10 percent, that would be a medical breakthrough. Our response rate was 100 percent, meaning researchers had a hard time believing it even after it had published in a peer-reviewed journal. Yet for the patients who got their sight back, it was a miracle. Not surprisingly, the higher the levels of omega-3 fatty acids used, the greater the extent of their vision improvement, and the faster it returned.

Of course, this doesn't mean you should start buying cases of fish oil in the health food store or supermarket. For one thing, it is probably high in PCBs. Second, it may be unsuitable for human consumption due to a high Totox level. And because you are going to need a lot of omega-3, you need exceptionally pure fish oil. You don't want a lot of PCBs and aldehydes and ketones in your body. (As I explained in Dirty Secret #3, aldehydes and ketones are toxic products of oxidation, besides generating the off odors associated with rancidity.)

If you can treat the brain, you can treat every other organ that is compromised by inflammation. To ensure you are taking enough omega-3 fatty acids and at the same time assure your doctor that you are not going to bleed to death (and you won't), you should check your AA/EPA ratio once a year.

You might be asking yourself: Would I do this for my own mother? Well, I did. My mother developed lung cancer at age 84 (she had stopped smoking forty years earlier). I told her I might not be able to stop the cancer, but I could guarantee that she would have no pain. This is always the great fear for cancer patients because, as the cancer spreads to other organs (especially the bone), it is usually accompanied by extraordinary pain that destroys all the dignity of life. To fulfill my promise, I gave her 40 grams of EPA and DHA per day. Although she died a year later, up to her last day of life, she was never in pain and was always in great spirits. That year gave everyone the chance to say all the things we wanted to say to her, retell the old family stories, and laugh at the same old jokes that we had shared for decades. It was a remarkable way to wrap up a lifetime of memories. These were all the things I didn't get a chance to share with my father when he died suddenly of a heart attack at age 53 nearly forty years earlier. She died in her sleep about a year after the cancer diagnosis when all of her organ systems failed simultaneously (due to the spread of the cancer). It is definitely the way I would want to end my life—in my own bed and with dignity.

What if you just want to live longer? One of the best ways to increase longevity is to increase the length of the telomeres attached to the end of your DNA. Their length is reduced each time the DNA is replicated. Once the telomeres reach a critical shortness, the DNA can no longer be replicated. Increasing the length of the telomeres increases the longevity of the DNA, which should translate into a longer life. In fact, the 2009 Nobel Prize in Medicine was awarded for understanding this relationship of telomere length and longevity. In 2013 one of those Nobel Prize winners for telomere research published a paper indicating that when subjects consumed more omega-3 fatty acids, the telomeres lengthened on their DNA.

How much omega-3 fatty acid was used at the highest dose? About 2.5 grams of omega-3 fatty acids per day. Not surprisingly, the highest dose used in that study is my minimum recommendation for the Mediterranean Zone. I suspect going to higher doses of omega-3 fatty acids will have an even greater impact on increasing telomere length. Just to emphasize the relationship of omega-3 fatty acids, telomere extension, and longevity, Harvard researchers also reported in 2013 that the higher the levels of omega-3 fatty acids in your blood, the longer you live.

These are just some of the reasons that you want to make sure you are taking enough omega-3 fatty acids to improve your memory, your sight, and your longevity.

Purified Polyphenol Extracts

There are more than eight thousand known polyphenols, but they are present in very low concentrations in fruits, whole grains, legumes, vegetables, and nuts. Unfortunately, whole grains contain a massive amount of glucose that will increase insulin levels and dramatically reduce many of the potential health benefits of polyphenols. So if your goal is the reduction of diet-induced inflammation, the use of whole grains as a source of polyphenols is probably not a great choice.

If you eat too many fruits and legumes, you can also stimulate insulin release. At least the levels of polyphenols per gram of carbohydrate are significantly higher than found in whole grains. Nonetheless, there is the risk of bingeing on fruits. This is not an uncommon observation in my experience, especially for women. It is why I usually recommend that women eat only one serving of fruit per day.

Nuts are low in carbohydrates, but they are incredibly rich sources of fat, so you can't simply gorge on nuts all day long. Although you wouldn't stimulate insulin that much by eating a lot of nuts, you will be taking in a massive amount of fat that has to be eventually stored in your fat cells. This leaves vegetables as the best overall source of polyphenols. Vegetables have the least impact on insulin and are virtually fat free. The only trouble is that you probably need to eat about two pounds of vegetables per day to get enough polyphenols to reach my recommendation of a minimum of consuming 1 gram of polyphenols per day.

Listed below are some levels of polyphenols in common foods known to have health benefits.

Food	Polyphenols per 100 g
Cocoa powder	3.3 grams
Blueberries	0.5 grams
Red wine	0.09 grams
Spinach	0.07 grams
Olive oil, extra-virgin	0.03 grams

This means getting 1 gram of polyphenols per day would require consuming more than 3 quarts of extra-virgin olive oil, or more than 10 glasses of red wine, or more than a cup of blueberries every day. Of course trying to consume 1 ounce of cocoa powder to get a gram of polyphenols takes incredible willpower due to its bitter taste (that's why they add sugar to it to make it palatable in dark chocolate bars).

Fortunately, polyphenols can be concentrated to a higher level by removing much of the non-polyphenol material to make it easier to achieve adequate levels in both the gut and the body. In the past, the primary methods of getting concentrated polyphenols in the traditional Mediterranean diet were drinking red wine, using extra-virgin olive oil, and drinking brewed extracts of certain beans rich in polyphenols (coffee and chocolate). All of these remain integral parts of the Mediterranean diet. Of course, there are some problems with each of these approaches.

Let's start with red wine. First, about one in seven who drink any form of alcohol will develop a dependence on it. Second, alcohol will negatively impact the brain by increasing the permeability of the blood-brain barrier with each drink, making it more likely that inflammatory mediators in the blood can enter the brain, thereby increasing neuroinflammation. Third, at some point (usually about two glasses of red wine per day), the negative consequences of the excess alcohol on the brain and the liver outweigh the health benefits of the extracted polyphenols in the red wine.

Another way of consuming a more concentrated form of polyphenols is extra-virgin olive oil. Olive oil is a fruit oil, not a seed oil. This means it is low in omega-6 fatty acids and rich in polyphenols. Because it is more expensive than vegetable oils, it has become an easy target for adulteration. Most of what is marketed as "extra-virgin" olive oil in the United States would be laughed at in Italy. However, even in Italy adulterated extra-virgin olive oil is a problem, and has been since the time of the Roman Empire, when official seals were placed on jugs of olive oil to prevent adulteration. However, there is a simple taste test for good olive oil. Take a teaspoon of olive oil and place it on the front of your tongue. It should taste like melted butter. This means it is very low in free fatty acids, which taste bitter. Then flip that olive oil to the back of your throat with your tongue. You should get a very peppery taste in your throat coupled with a strong urge to cough. That comes from the polyphenols. Only if the olive oil passes both tests can it be considered good quality. About 98 percent of "extra-virgin" olive oil sold in America fails to meet both of these two tests.

Finally, both unprocessed coffee and cocoa beans are rich in polyphenols, but the use of fermentation and roasting to release more flavors from the beans destroys most of the polyphenols. Nonetheless, they are still bitter. That's why people add both sugar and milk to dark coffee (think Frappuccino) and baker's chocolate (think candy bars).

Of course, you could add large amounts of spices, which are very rich sources of polyphenols, to every meal. At low levels, spices add flavor. Unfortunately, to get higher levels of polyphenols, they become a source of bitterness.

How do you get high levels of polyphenols without eating a massive amount of vegetables (at least to American tastes) and without adding inedible amounts of spices to your meals? One answer is purified polyphenol extracts. You have to extract them from natural sources and then purify them through a multi-step process of dehydration, followed by alcohol extraction, and then removing the alcohol and finally separating all the other non-polyphenol material using gigantic columns packed with specialized absorbents. It is a long and expensive process, but the end result is well worth it.

Is there potentially the "best of the best" when it comes to such purified polyphenols? Although the goal is to have as many different types of polyphenols in your diet (that's why you should be eating primarily a wide variety of vegetables), supplementing with purified polyphenol extracts means you have to make some educated choices. In my opinion, if you had to choose only one polyphenol class, I would put my money on delphinidins.

You may have never heard of this class of polyphenols, but you probably have consumed them. They are found in red wines, blueberries, and dark bitter chocolate. However, the highest concentration of delphinidins is found in the maqui berry, which grows only in the mountains of the Patagonian region of Chile that is very close to Antarctica. The combination of cold temperature, exposure to ozone (the ozone layer is very thin at the South Pole), and chilling winds coming off the Antarctic Ocean provide a hostile environment that the maqui berry responds to by an overproduction of delphinidins to protect the plant from the severe conditions of its environment.

Delphinidins have a unique structure compared to other polyphenols. As a result they are (1) more water soluble, which increases the likelihood of absorption by body, and (2) have a much less bitter taste compared to other highly purified polyphenol extracts, which means they are more easily incorporated into food products or meals.

The water solubility of delphinidins also appears to enhance their ability to activate the "enzyme of life" (AMP kinase). This enzyme is also a master genetic switch that controls metabolism in every cell and, in particular, increases the production of chemical energy from dietary calories. If you are consuming adequate levels of polyphenols to activate this enzyme, then you can get significant increase in chemical energy (ATP) production. This means you need far fewer calories to maintain high levels of physical and mental energy. If you eat fewer calories, you slow down the aging process (in addition to losing weight). And if you use the Mediterranean Zone as a blueprint to balance those reduced number of incoming calories, you slow the aging process even more.

Purified delphinidins are probably the only class of polyphenols that don't have a bitter taste and at the same time are completely water soluble. If you add one capsule of purified delphinidins to water, you instantly get a glass that looks like the richest red wine but has a taste similar to water. In fact, that glass of delphinidin "wine" would have twice the polyphenols as a glass of the most robust red wine. There is great potential of using such a delphinidin "wine" as the ultimate energy drink. If you really want to drink of a glass of red wine, then add one capsule of purified delphinidins to it and turn it into "super wine" with three times the polyphenols as the original glass of red wine. Of course, adding the same delphinidin extract to vodka or gin takes an alcoholic beverage with no health benefits and turns either of those refined alcoholic beverages into a relatively healthy drink (at least in terms of polyphenol content).

Historically, the Mapuche, an indigenous people of southern Chile, were the only Native Americans in South America not to be conquered by Europeans. Their warriors were reputed to have tremendous stamina that allowed them to constantly thwart the Europeans, who obviously had superior weapons technology. Perhaps not surprisingly, maqui berries were an integral part of their diet.

Over time, the use of maqui berries was forgotten in Chile. The interest in them was revived only a few years ago by the Chilean government, which was looking for new sources of value-added products to export. The Chilean government has invested a lot of money on optimization of the maqui berry by supporting high-quality agricultural and clinical research. Part of that research has indicated that high levels of delphinidins significantly stimulate the enzyme of life. This would explain the remarkable stamina of the Mapuche warriors. It also means that high enough concentrations of the delphinidins may also provide significant weight-loss potential, because if you can generate adequate levels of chemical energy to keep the body going, then you can consume fewer calories without fatigue (such as the Mapuche warriors). If you are consuming fewer calories, then you will lose weight. That same reduction in calories also slows down the aging process. Increased weight loss without fatigue and a decreased rate of aging is not a bad combination.

As with all natural products, you still have to consume enough foods containing delphinidins to get these benefits. You could drink red wine or eat bitter dark chocolate to obtain high levels of delphinidins, but you would probably need to consume about five hundred bottles of red wine per day or eat a hundred bars of dark extremely bitter chocolate (containing 100 percent cocoa) to get a therapeutic level of this unique polyphenol. Alternatively, you might consume 5 pounds of blueberries on a daily basis. None of these are likely to happen. The fourth option is to take one or two capsules of a highly purified delphinidin extract. That is more likely to occur in the real world.

Of course, the question is how much can you safely take? Basic safety research done by the Chilean government has shown that the purified delphinidin extract from the maqui berry is incredibly safe, with a toxicity approaching that of water. In fact, a highly purified extract of the maqui berry (Delphinol) was recently granted Generally Regarded as Safe (GRAS) status by the FDA, meaning it is safe to be added to food products. To my knowledge, no other purified polyphenol has reached that level of safety testing, which means they have to be sold as nutritional supplements (meaning buyer beware), not as GRAS food additives.

Can you take too much of a purified maqui extract? It's highly unlikely, because most delphinidins stay in the gut to promote the maintenance of a healthy balance of microbes, and only a very small percentage of the delphinidins actually enter the bloodstream. Nonetheless, their benefits are very dose dependent. At low levels of delphinidin intake (about 50 to 150 mg per day), they function as a powerful anti-oxidant (as you might expect, given that they exist to protect the maqui berry from radiation coming from a depleted ozone layer). At increased concentrations (150 to 300 mg per day), they begin to inhibit of the master genetic switch of cellular inflammation. Finally, at still higher levels (greater than 300 mg per day), delphinidins begin to activate the enzyme of life, leading to a slowing of the aging process.

Taking purified maqui extracts rich in delphinidins may represent the easiest way to slow the aging process as well as simultaneously impress your friends when you turn water into delphinidin wine.

PART II

The Science of Polyphenols

7

Polyphenols:
The Next Essential Nutrients

I knew very little about polyphenols when I wrote *The Zone* in 1995. My interest at the time was trying to reduce insulin production by maintaining a lower glycemic load in the diet. It just happened that low-glycemic load carbohydrates were also rich in polyphenols. It wasn't until much later that I realized there was a lot more to polyphenols than simply imparting color to fruits and vegetables.

As a science, nutrition is still in its infancy. We know that calories are converted to the chemical energy that allows us to survive and function. We also know that the balance of carbohydrates, protein, and fat in the diet (via the hormones they generate) governs the efficiency of our metabolism. And we also know that dietary protein and fats contain certain amino acids and fatty acids that are essential for life and must be supplied by our diet. In addition to essential amino and fatty acids, our diet also has to provide our body with the essential vitamins and minerals it can't synthesize on its own.

I believe that in a few years polyphenols, which cannot be synthesized by our bodies, will also be included in this category of essential nutrients. The reason that it is taking so long to come to that conclusion is that polyphenols work in more subtle ways than other essential nutrients. Only recently with new breakthroughs in molecular biology have we been able to study their unique effects on human physiology. Their importance to human health has only become more evident as increasing industrialization of our foods has resulted in a dramatic reduction in their nutritional content—and our overall wellness.

There are interesting parallels between the realization of the importance of polyphenols and vitamins. One of the first industrialized foods was white rice. Removing the outer husk of brown rice to produce white rice created a much longer shelf life. The unintended consequence in the refining of brown rice was the creation of a deficiency in vitamin B_1 (thiamine), leading to beriberi, a disorder that impairs cardiovascular and nerve function with symptoms that include tingling and numbness in extremities, fatigue, and loss of appetite. Subsequently, it was discovered that a trace ingredient in the outer husk on grains of rice quickly cured the disease. That trace ingredient was vitamin B_1. Although vitamin deficiencies are easily observed and can be rapidly corrected, deficiencies in polyphenols (which are found in small amounts in brown rice but in larger amounts in brightly colored fruits and vegetables) are far subtler because they are manifested only with the development of inflammatory diseases, and our knowledge of the molecular biology of inflammation remains relatively primitive.

Although you may not be aware of the scientific evidence for the health benefits of polyphenols, you've probably heard stories about them that have been told through history without knowing that polyphenols were central to their content.

Three Wise Men
The three wise men who brought gifts to the newborn Christ child in the Christian Bible came bearing not only gold, but also spices—frankincense and myrrh—which were worth far more than gold at that time because of their ability to preserve food. After all, having a lot of gold wasn't worth too much if you were dying of food poisoning.

The Aphrodisiac Secrets of Chocolate
One of the most sought-after treasures of Central and South America by the Spanish conquistadors after gold and silver was chocolate. It was prized for both its medical and aphrodisiac benefits. It was said that Montezuma

would have a couple of stiff drinks of bitter chocolate before visiting his bevy of wives. That benefit was not lost on the Spanish nobility.

An Apple a Day Keeps the Doctor Away

It's certainly not the water or the sugars or even the fiber in the apple that does the job. Remove all of those items from the apple, and you get a very small amount of powder that is extremely bitter to the taste. The powder contains the apple's polyphenols, which provide the real nutritional benefit that keeps the doctor away.

Parsley, Sage, Rosemary, and Thyme

Other than being the title of a popular Simon and Garfunkel song, these spices have among the highest levels of polyphenols and were considered essential for food preservation in medieval times.

You are probably aware of other food products rich in polyphenols. For example, we constantly hear about the benefits of red wine, and yet no one talks about the health benefits of vodka. That's because there are none. The intensity of the color of wine is critical in providing those health benefits. Red wine contains ten times more polyphenols than white wine. (At least white wine contains more polyphenols than vodka.) This may explain why red wine is the primary wine consumed in the Mediterranean region.

Polyphenols are found in nuts, vegetables, fruits, legumes, and even whole grains, but each of these food products has increasing levels of carbohydrates that will increase insulin secretion. Nuts have the lowest glycemic response because they are primarily fat, which has no effect on the glycemic load. (Yes, you could eat only nuts and consume of a lot of polyphenols, but it is very easy to over-consume them and take the fat content of the Mediterranean Zone well beyond the "dash of fat" level.) Vegetables have the next lowest glycemic load, followed by fruits. Whole grains have a very high glycemic load, almost as high as white carbohydrates (bread, pasta, rice, and potatoes). So why do you hear so much about the benefits of whole grains? Because they contain polyphenols, but the potential health benefits of the polyphenols in whole grains are significantly reduced by the powerful insulin-stimulating properties of carbohydrates in those whole grains.

If you want the greatest health benefits from polyphenols without excess fat or insulin secretion, then most of your carbohydrates should come from colorful, non-starchy vegetables, with limited amounts of fruit. As for the whole grains, they simply supply too much glucose considering the amount of polyphenols you get.

These foods are not the only sources of polyphenols in the American diet. The primary source of polyphenols for most Americans is coffee. Another source in the American diet is chocolate.

Of course, everyone loves chocolate, but the polyphenols in it make unsweetened chocolate incredibly bitter. Montezuma may have taken his chocolate unsweetened, but the Europeans had a taste for sweeter stuff. To make chocolate more palatable, manufacturers add increasing amounts of sugar. If it's a little sugar, it's called dark chocolate. Add even more sugar and milk, and it's a milk chocolate candy bar. Of course if you use "Dutch process" cocoa, which sounds elegant but really means it has been treated with sodium hydroxide to destroy most of the polyphenols, then you have a much better tasting source of chocolate. Not surprisingly, most commercial chocolate products use Dutch process chocolate and, as a result, many of the potential health benefits of the cocoa polyphenols have been largely destroyed. Any benefits of the remaining polyphenols are further compromised by the added sugar.

The polyphenols in wine, especially red wine, are just as bitter as those that naturally occur in cocoa. Let a glass of red wine totally evaporate and then taste the residue in the bottom of the glass. It's incredibly bitter. The alcohol in the wine not only extracts the polyphenols very effectively from grapes but also dampens the taste receptors on the tongue (which are very sensitive to bitter-tasting ingredients) so you can't taste how bitter those healthy polyphenols really are. Consider red wine to simply be a very efficient grape polyphenol delivery system.

The richest sources of polyphenols, however, are spices. Throughout history spices have been valued not only for their culinary and medicinal uses, but also for their ability to preserve food by reducing oxidation. Remember your grade school history lessons? America was "discovered" by explorers looking for a shorter route to the Far East, the source of many prized spices.

Obviously, polyphenols have an important purpose for plants; otherwise they wouldn't devote so much of their valuable energy to making them. One obvious reason is that plants are constantly exposed to ionizing radiation from the sun. Polyphenols are powerful anti-oxidants that neutralize the free radicals formed by constant sun exposure. Another reason is that polyphenols are powerful anti-microbial agents. Unlike humans, plants don't have a sophisticated array of immunological defense systems to defend themselves against microbiological attack; the presence of polyphenols is their primary biochemical defense weapon.

Why is this important to humans? The polyphenols in our diet play a critical role in maintaining an optimal balance between the good and bad microbes that make up our digestive system—all four pounds of them. Once we take polyphenols out of the human diet, we become a much easier target for pathological microbes and their toxins to enter the bloodstream, causing increased cellular inflammation throughout the body. Increased inflammation accelerates the development of chronic disease and speeds up the aging process. The most extreme case of microbe-induced inflammation is septic shock, with a mortality rate of nearly 50 percent.

One reason it is increasingly difficult to consume a sufficient amount polyphenols from our food is genetic engineering, the old-fashioned kind that is the result of thousands of years of crossbreeding to make fruits and vegetables tastier. For example, wild Italian strawberries are quite small and bitter. The strawberries you buy in the supermarket are large and sweet because they have been bred to dilute out the (bitter) polyphenols with sugar. Good news for your taste buds; bad news for your health. In addition, the use of herbicides and pesticides reduce the levels of polyphenols in plants. The less the plant has to work to fight off microbes, the more it diverts its energy to make more sugar—and fewer polyphenols. This is why conventionally raised fruits and vegetables are picture perfect: big, with no bruises or defects. Organic produce, on the other hand, often looks like it's been in a street fight. The lack of uniform color and shape, the lumps and scars on their surface, are the collateral damage of polyphenols fighting off pests and microbes in the absence of pesticides. It's also an indication of the higher levels of polyphenols in organic fruits and vegetables.

Another important reason polyphenols should be considered essential nutrients is because we are only partially human. We are really composite organisms with ten times more microbes (primarily bacteria) inside our bodies than human cells. Most of the bacteria in our bodies reside in the gut and especially in the colon. If you take into account relative contributions to the amount of DNA in our body (including the bacteria in the gut), then only 1 percent of our total DNA can be considered human. Gut bacteria—and how polyphenols can modify their composition in the gut—may be more valuable to our health than vitamins. In fact, most of the polyphenols that we ingest are used primarily to manage the 100 trillion bacteria in our gut.

To get enough polyphenols to maintain optimal health, I usually recommend that you consume about 1 gram on a daily basis. This means that controlling the balance of our gut microbes requires eating a lot of vegetables and fruits. The levels of polyphenols in fruit is about 0.2 percent of their total weight. The polyphenol content in vegetables is even less (about 0.1 percent of their total weight). This means you have to eat either 1 pound of fruit or 2 pounds of vegetables per day to reach my recommended level of consuming 1 gram of polyphenols. The polyphenol content of unsweetened cocoa powder is much greater at 3.5 percent of the total weight, but most individuals are not going to be eating a lot of unsweetened cocoa powder.

When you consider these numbers, all of a sudden the likelihood of achieving good health with adequate levels of polyphenols begins to seem like mission impossible. Of course, other polyphenols can be added to your diet with the liberal consumption of spices, red wine, and extra-virgin olive oil, all key components of the Mediterranean diet. Or you can add polyphenols by supplementing your diet with purified polyphenol extracts, a more high-tech solution.

The first step in consuming enough polyphenols is finding sources you like to eat. That's a lot easier in Mediterranean countries where fruits and vegetables still make up a significant portion of their standard diet. Coffee is the primary source of polyphenols for Americans, and our consumption of fruits and vegetables is rather pathetic. The average American consumes about 450 mg of polyphenols per day with most of that coming from coffee. (Each cup provides about 100 mg of polyphenols, and average consumption is about 3 cups per day.)

The power of polyphenols is the combination of the amount you consume as well as the amount that is actually absorbed by your body. At low levels, they are powerful anti-bacterial agents in the gut, but very little is absorbed by the body. At higher levels, they act as anti-oxidants and anti-inflammatory agents within the body. At still higher levels, they become anti-aging agents that can significantly increase longevity. Unfortunately, the polyphenol levels that the average American absorbs on a daily basis are way below the minimums needed for demonstrating a significant improvement in health. This is why following the Mediterranean Zone has such profound benefits in such a short period of time, because we are consuming much higher levels of polyphenols that have multi-factorial benefits on health.

In the next chapters, I will discuss each of the areas in which polyphenols can profoundly impact human health.

8

Polyphenols and Gut Health

One reason polyphenols are so critical to human health is because we actually have two brains in our body: the brain inside our skull that contains our personality and cognitive thinking, and the brain we never think about, the one found in our digestive system. Unlike our nicely contained thinking brain, our second brain is smelly, slimy, and messy. Yet these two brains are in constant communication with each other, and the levels and types of bacteria in the gut have an important role to play in this communication. Keeping those rowdy 100 trillion bacteria in line means maintaining a healthy level of good bacteria in the gut—a primary job of polyphenols. This is why improved gut health is one of the main benefits of following the Mediterranean Zone. As you increase the levels of polyphenols in your diet, you also increase one of your primary dietary defenses for managing inflammation in both your digestive brain and thinking brain.

We have been co-evolving with bacteria since the beginning of our species some 200,000 years ago. Of the millions of different bacteria in the world, only about five hundred to a thousand different types actually reside in our gut. Probably more than 99 percent of the 100 trillion bacteria consist of thirty to forty types of bacteria. This indicates that the composition of our gut microbes is not the result of some random process.

The 100 trillion residents in our gut can be either friends or foes. I say *friends* because they can help digest carbohydrates that are not easily absorbed (unabsorbed carbohydrates cause diarrhea), produce certain vitamins, train the immune system in the intestine to be on alert for really bad (pathogenic) bacteria that may enter into the digestive system, and take a defensive position on the surface of the gut to prevent bad bacteria from getting a foothold. It's a great symbiotic arrangement for both the good bacteria and us. The chosen bacteria get a safe environment with lots of nutrients, and in return they provide us real protection from their potentially dangerous microbial cousins.

Since about 30 percent of the total solid component of our stools is composed of dead bacteria, to maintain this symbiotic relationship, the gut microbiological community needs to be continually stimulated to grow and replenish itself. Polyphenols act as the ultimate prebiotics in stimulating friendly bacterial growth. It is the more rapid growth of the colonic bacteria in the gut that increases stool size, not merely the fiber content of the diet.

Polyphenols also act as anti-microbial agents against bad bacteria (as well as viruses, fungi, and parasites). The bottom line is that as long as you have a constant dietary intake of a lot of polyphenols, you are going to have good gut health, and that translates into improved overall health. Unfortunately, pharmaceutical progress can get in the way of a good thing.

One of the gifts of pharmaceutical progress has been the advent of antibiotics. If there was ever a wonder drug, it must be antibiotics. In fact, they work so well that the drug industry no longer likes them because they are both inexpensive and are needed for only short periods of time (resulting in fewer profits to the drug companies). In the 1950s farmers discovered that if they gave low levels of antibiotics to their cattle, pigs, and chickens, their livestock would grow faster. The increased growth was because the animals were getting fatter. Unsurprisingly, more than 80 percent of antibiotics produced today are used for veterinary purposes as opposed to treating human disease. No one thought too much of this until the obesity epidemic in America began nearly forty years ago. Only recently, with the advancement of genetic techniques, has it been possible to investigate the connection between bacterial composition in the gut and obesity and other chronic diseases.

It is known that obese individuals have a different bacteria composition in their gut than lean individuals. That is only a correlation with obesity, not a definite cause. However, it is known that obesity is caused by cellular inflammation in the fat cells. Could it be that a poor composition of bacteria in the gut might further increase cellular inflammation in those fat cells and facilitate its spread to other organs in the body? Here I think the answer is a definite yes.

However, it takes two to tango. For cellular inflammation to spread, you need the combination of not only (1) insufficient levels of good gut bacteria, but also (2) increased cellular inflammation in the membranes lining the gut. Just as you have two brains, you also have two skins on your body. There is the outer skin that is impermeable and keeps the microbes from the outer world from invading the body. Your second skin is far more complex. This is the lining of the gut. It not only has to prevent any bacteria from entering the body, but also must be a dynamic filter to allow digested nutrients to enter and at the same time to communicate (via hormones) the realtime nutrient status in the gut to the brain in your skull. If communication between the gut and the brain is compromised, then your brain is constantly led to believe that there are not enough nutrients in the digestive system—and it keeps sending signals for you to eat more food. The lack of satiety coming from disruption in gut-and-brain communication is also accompanied by increased cellular inflammation throughout the body, which leads to the development of obesity, chronic diseases such as diabetes, and accelerating the onset of Alzheimer's.

To understand how this happens, you have to understand a little about toll-like receptors. I will explain more of this in greater detail in the Appendices, but here is a short overview. Toll-like receptors are molecules that act as biological sensors to detect bacterial fragments. These sensors occupy the cell surface of every living cell in the body. Although these toll-like receptors are ancient, our knowledge of them is recent. In fact, the 2011 Nobel Prize in Medicine was awarded for understanding their impact on human health.

We have ten unique toll-like receptors, each capable of recognizing different microbial fragments. If a microbial fragment, leaked from the gut into the bloodstream, activates any of the receptors, cells prepare for a potential microbial attack by immediately increasing the expression of inflammatory proteins from its nucleus containing your DNA. All of this is done through the most primitive part of our immune system, the innate immune system. Continued activation of these toll-like receptors by leaking bacterial fragments from the gut into the bloodstream results in the generation of chronic low levels of cellular inflammation. This disrupts hormonal signals, especially of insulin, and can lead to insulin resistance. Once insulin resistance sets in, it begins a downward spiral effectively resulting in obesity, diabetes, and acceleration of other chronic inflammatory diseases (such as Alzheimer's).

As the levels of good bacteria decrease in the gut (because of lack of adequate levels of polyphenols in the diet), more pathogenic (really bad) bacteria have the opportunity to enter the bloodstream. You can decrease the level of good bacteria in your gut by (1) frequent courses of antibiotic treatments from your physician, (2) ingesting animal products that were fed a steady diet of antibiotics, and (3) by not consuming enough polyphenols. Add to this an increasing intake of omega-6 fatty acids and decrease in omega-3 fatty acids in the general diet, and you are virtually assured the lining of the gut will be inflamed, giving rise to gaps in an otherwise strong biological barrier to prevent the entry of bad bacteria and large, undigested proteins. This is what is called leaky gut syndrome. Now more bacteria (as well as other intact dietary proteins such as those found in gluten-containing or dairy products) are able to enter into the bloodstream and the levels of cellular inflammation are increased throughout the body. When that happens, you gain weight, accelerate the development of chronic disease, and age faster.

Obviously, your primary dietary strategies to lose weight, maintain wellness, and age at a slower rate have to be based on maintaining a healthy gut. This means eating about 2 pounds of vegetables per day. This isn't as hard as it seems. For example, two pounds of vegetables might be composed of two large red peppers, one large red onion, ½ pound of asparagus, ¼ pound of broccoli, and ¼ pound of cauliflower. Cut them up and roast them with a little extra-virgin olive oil at night and then eat them throughout the next day. Alternatively, you could use a couple bags of steamed frozen vegetables. Their preparation takes only about 6 to 8 minutes in a microwave. You can also supplement your diet with a daily glass of red wine. One glass of red wine has the polyphenol equivalent of eating about 100 mg of polyphenols. If you've already done the math, you've figured out that if you drank ten glasses of red wine per day, you wouldn't need to eat any vegetables at all. Good math, but bad biochemistry since that level of alcohol wipes out virtually all of the health benefits of the polyphenols.

Getting enough polyphenols for gut health requires some dietary discipline, but keep in mind your health is one of the things money can't buy. And much of your future health will depend on controlling cellular inflammation in the stinky and slimy second brain known as the gut. Every time you sit down to a meal, you have an opportunity to invest in your future health. Following the Mediterranean Zone makes that investment strategy easy to follow. Furthermore, if you mess up with one meal, the guidelines of the Mediterranean Zone tell you exactly what you need to do to get right back into the Zone.

9

Polyphenols
and Oxidative Stress

We often think of free radicals as dangerous to our health, but free radicals, such as inflammation, are critical to support life. Free radicals allow you to convert dietary calories (food) into chemical energy, create hormones and other complex molecules, and provide the most powerful agents we have to kill invading microbes. However, unless you manage the levels of these constantly generated free radicals, they will start attacking normal tissue, and you will age at a faster rate. The scientific name for such excess free radical production is oxidative stress. To maintain optimal health, polyphenols are critical for controlling the level of free radicals.

Our immune cells (neutrophils and macrophages) make a wide array of free radicals, including a biological form of Clorox known as hypochlorite. In addition to this biological bleach (which kills microbes very effectively), there are other types of free radicals generated by our immune cells, such as:

Hydroxyl (OH•)
Peroxyl (ROH•)

Peroxynitrite (ONOO•)

Superoxide anion (O_2•)

The one thing that these free radicals all have in common is an unpaired electron (•) that hates to be alone and will go out of its way to extract another electron to keep it company. This extraction of electrons from other biomolecules is one of the key steps in metabolism that allows the synthesis of very complex molecules. If free radical generation is not constrained, then the oxidative stress that is generated leads to DNA fragmentation and cell death. Polyphenols sacrifice themselves by donating one of their hydrogen atoms to the free radical to effectively quench excess free radicals, reducing the levels of oxidative stress within the cell.

The immune cells that generate these free radicals come from otherwise benign white cells circulating in your bloodstream. Once the innate immune system senses the existence of microbial fragments, a complex process is started that transforms the white blood cells happily circulating in your bloodstream into the cellular dogs of war (neutrophils and macrophages) to do battle against microbes. Just like radiation coming from X-rays (or an atomic bomb blast), these free radicals generated by neutrophils and macrophages are killers. Eventually, these biological rogue warriors must be called off during the resolution phase of the inflammatory response, which is described in greater detail in the Appendices.

The resolution phase of inflammation shuts down the inflammatory attack by the synthesis of powerful hormones called resolvins, derived from omega-3 fatty acids (EPA and DHA). Without adequate levels of omega-3 fatty acids in the diet, the resolution phase of inflammation will be compromised. These resolvins are critical for causing the destruction of the newly generated neutrophils and macrophages and returning the body back to equilibrium. If the initial inflammatory signal is too strong, or if the resolution response for turning off the initial inflammatory response is too weak, then these immune cells continue to hang around, spewing out a continual stream of free radicals.

Another source of free radicals is the constant need to convert dietary calories into chemical energy (usually the molecule adenosine triphosphate, or ATP). The amount of calories you consume doesn't count as much as the efficiency of their conversion into ATP. Without adequate levels of ATP, your cells can't function efficiently to maintain your metabolism and cellular renewal, nor can you maintain enough energy for the physical demands on your body, such as walking or running. The conversion of dietary calories into ATP takes place in the mitochrondria found in every cell in the body. The process of making ATP requires the generation of a lot of free radicals, and invariably some of these free radicals escape. Obviously, the fewer the calories you eat, the fewer free radicals you make. This is one of the reasons calorie restriction (without malnutrition) slows down the rate of aging. Restrict calories and add more polyphenols to your diet, and you can live even longer.

The strength of an anti-oxidant molecule can be measured by its ability to neutralize free radicals. This can be quantified in a test tube to provide a quantitative ranking system known as the oxygen radical absorption capacity (ORAC), which estimates the potential of a given amount of a food product to act as an anti-oxidant. It has been shown that the ORAC value of a food ingredient is correlated with the levels of polyphenols in the same ingredient. Some polyphenols are best at neutralizing free radicals in the water-soluble environment (such as in your blood) whereas others work best in the lipid environment (as in lipoprotein particles or in cell membranes). Therefore what you need is a total ORAC value that represents the combination of both types of anti-oxidant activities. The higher the total ORAC level of a food ingredient, the better its potential ability to act as an anti-oxidant.

Listed below are some of the total ORAC values of common foods. A more complete list can be found in Appendix G.

Food Item	Serving Size	ORAC/100 g
Apple	100 g	3,049
Broccoli	100 g	1,510
Pumpernickel bread	100 g	1,963

Looking at the chart above, it is not clear why eating broccoli is a better dietary choice than pumpernickel bread. It is only apparent when you take into account the amount of carbohydrates you are simultaneously ingesting to obtain those anti-oxidative polyphenols. So let's redo the same table and see what food item provides the greatest amount of anti-oxidants with the least amount of absorbable carbohydrates (defined as total carbohydrates minus fiber).

Food Item	Serving Size	ORAC/100 g	ORAC/g Carbohydrate
Apple	100 g	3,049	282
Broccoli	100 g	1,510	356
Pumpernickel bread	100 g	1,963	48

As you can see above, the levels of polyphenols per gram of carbohydrate is seven times greater in broccoli than pumpernickel bread. This means you would be consuming seven times more carbohydrates by eating pumpernickel bread instead of the broccoli to get the same levels of anti-oxidants. To make this comparison even more compelling, the carbohydrates in the pumpernickel bread (as with all whole grains) are composed of virtually 100 percent glucose, whereas the carbohydrates in fruits and vegetables have lower levels of glucose and higher levels of fructose. The more glucose you consume, the more insulin you secrete. And if you are consuming a lot of omega-6 fatty acids at the same time, you will be generating more cellular inflammation. Frankly, it just isn't worth the hormonal hassle to eat whole grain breads and cereals to get the necessary levels of polyphenols you need to reduce oxidative stress.

I can do the same type of calculations for herbs and spices using dried rosemary as an example.

Food Item	Serving Size	ORAC/100 g	ORAC/g Carbohydrate
Rosemary, dried	100 g	165,280	7,702

Obviously, no one is going to eat 100 grams (which is 3.5 ounces or nearly 10 tablespoons of dried rosemary), but you can quickly see that rosemary (such as most spices) is a tremendous source of anti-oxidants with very little accompanying carbohydrate.

Here is another problem: It does not matter how many polyphenols you consume, but how many of those get into the bloodstream to exert their anti-oxidant actions. Only 2 to 20 percent of consumed polyphenols actually enters into blood. Once a polyphenol enters the blood, it is rapidly metabolized so that it can be excreted. A polyphenol is at its peak level usually within two hours of consumption, then is rapidly metabolized and is completely eliminated from the body, usually through the urine, within twelve hours. This means that virtually all the polyphenols consumed in a meal are out of your body within twelve hours. To maintain a constant level of these powerful anti-oxidants in the blood you either have to have a lot of colorful carbohydrates at every meal or take a very large amount of purified polyphenols several times a day.

So how do you know if the polyphenols you are consuming are actually doing you much good? You really have to look at indirect markers of reducing oxidative stress. One of these markers is the level of oxidized LDL.

For more than forty years, the medical community has been misled in thinking the level of total LDL cholesterol is a driving force for the development of heart disease. Actually, a major culprit in heart disease is not plain old normal LDL particles, but oxidized LDL particles. Oxidized LDL particles are able to sneak into the cell through a backdoor pathway, whereas normal LDL particles cannot. Thus much of the accumulated cholesterol in an atherosclerotic plaque is composed of oxidized LDL particles. Until recently, measuring oxidized LDL directly was very difficult and as a result, calculating total LDL cholesterol has been unknowingly used as a surrogate marker for oxidized LDL without anyone realizing it. The real relationship between heart disease and cholesterol was really one based on the levels of oxidized LDL particles.

Statins became the most profitable drugs in history because while they were lowering normal LDL cholesterol they were also lowering the levels of oxidized LDL. But with statins it was a case of throwing the baby out with the bathwater since you need normal, non-oxidized LDL to deliver adequate levels of cholesterol to the brain to maintain cognitive function. This is why one of the major side effects of statins is memory loss. Polyphenols, on the other hand, can directly reduce the levels of oxidized LDL without reducing LDL cholesterol. That's one of the reasons adherence to the traditional Mediterranean diet simultaneously reduces heart disease and improves cognitive function in the brain.

The dual power of polyphenols for both heart and brain health was demonstrated using high-dose polyphenols derived from blueberries in two separate clinical studies in 2010. One study at the University of Oklahoma demonstrated a statistically significant 30 percent reduction in levels of oxidized LDL. The other study at the University of Cincinnati demonstrated significant improvement in cognition in older adults with impaired memory. It should be noted that delphinidins are one of the major classes of polyphenols in blueberries. If blueberries are good, then purified polyphenol extracts from the maqui berry I described earlier should be better as they are fourteen times more concentrated in delphinidins than blueberries. It appears that if you consume enough polyphenols (and delphinidins look like a really good choice), then your likelihood of heart disease and Alzheimer's should be reduced.

So how many ORAC units do you need to consume on a daily basis to get a sufficient amount of polyphenols? If you consume the recommended five to nine servings of fruits and vegetables per day, which virtually no one in America does, you would probably get about 3,000 to 5,000 ORAC units per day. A study at Tufts Medical School in 1996 indicated if you increased your intake to ten servings of common fruits and vegetables per day, you would consume about 6,000 ORAC units per day. Even though you are doubling the dietary intake of polyphenols, the anti-oxidant levels in the blood increase by only about 10 percent because most polyphenols have a very low absorption rate by the body. Although this may seem like a case of diminishing returns, if you consume enough polyphenols on a daily basis, the payoff in reducing the oxidative stress on the body is remarkable. What I generally recommend is the daily consumption of about 10,000 ORAC units to reduce oxidative stress. To reach that, you will probably need to supplement your consumption of colorful carbohydrates with perhaps a glass of red wine, adding a couple of tablespoons of authentic extra-virgin olive oil, or taking highly purified polyphenol extracts in a pill or liquid form.

However, what truly makes polyphenols unique in addition to their ability to neutralize free radicals is their ability to increase the production of additional powerful anti-oxidant proteins by binding them to a specialized gene transcription factor. Every cell contains unique proteins called gene transcription factors that let the cell fine-tune the expression of its gene responses to its immediate environment by turning unique sets of genes on or off. The one such gene transcription factor activated by polyphenols is known as Nrf2. Once it is activated, it can accelerate the synthesis of a wide array of additional powerful anti-oxidative proteins. These proteins not only effectively neutralize free radicals but also regenerate other anti-oxidant molecules. Polyphenols should really be viewed as super anti-oxidants because they're able to quench free radicals very effectively on their own, but they also have the ability to enlist the synthesis of new anti-oxidant enzymes so that you can continue your lifelong struggle against oxidative stress.

Can you take too many anti-oxidants? Of course you can, especially if they are the kind of anti-oxidants that easily enter into the blood, such as vitamin E, beta-carotene, and vitamin C. This is especially true if you are taking chemotherapeutic drugs that rely on increased free radical generation caused by the cancer drug to kill the cancer cells by causing fragmentation of its DNA. Likewise, too many anti-oxidants in the blood can blunt the ability of the immune system to destroy invading microbes as well as potentially creating pro-oxidant effects. However, most people have enough trouble eating my recommended daily servings of fruits and vegetables to get the necessary polyphenols they need. That's why your grandmother told your parents that they couldn't leave the dinner table until they had finished all their vegetables. Who knew that Grandma was the cutting edge of twenty-first-century biotechnology to reduce oxidative stress?

10

Polyphenols and Longevity

As important as polyphenols are in reducing excess free radicals and oxidative stress, their most important property may be their ability to slow the rate of aging.

Who doesn't want to live longer? One of the first indications that it was possible to extend your life through diet came from the writings of Luigi Cornaro, a Venetian nobleman, who lived in the fifteenth century. Finding himself near death at age 35 because of his rich dietary lifestyle, he went on a strict calorie-restricted diet consisting of an egg yolk, some vegetable soup, small amounts of locally grown fruits and vegetables, and a very small amount of coarse, unrefined bread, as well as three glasses of red wine per day. He wrote his first anti-aging book, *The Sure and Certain Method of Attaining a Long and Healthful Life,* at age 83 and his third anti-aging book at age 95. He died at age 99. At the end of his life he was still mentally sharp and physically active.

Nearly four hundred years later in 1935 Clive McCay demonstrated that calorie restriction could dramatically prolong the lifespan of rats. Since then the benefits of calorie restriction have been reproduced in a wide number of other animal species. Luigi Cornaro's highly restrictive caloric diet can be estimated to have been between 800 and 1,000 calories per day, hardly enough calories to generate the chemical energy a human needs to live. But obviously Luigi did a pretty good job for ninety-nine years. Is it possible that the polyphenols in the red wine also helped? The answer may be yes.

What we usually term as aging may be viewed as the combined consequences of either increased cellular inflammation and/or decreased metabolic efficiency. Thus, anything that reduces inflammation or increases metabolic efficacy should extend longevity. To find that connection, you have to return to the subject of gene transcription factors. Among the unique ability of polyphenols to reduce oxidative stress, they also activate other gene transcription factors in our cells that can help us to live longer by increasing metabolic efficacy and decreasing inflammation.

One of those factors is an enzyme known as AMP kinase. It is called the enzyme of life because it senses the chemical energy levels in the cell and then adjusts the metabolism of the cell to maximize energy (adenosine triphosphate, or ATP) production. AMP kinase is also a master genetic switch for increasing the efficacy of the metabolism in every one of the 10 trillion cells in the body. Once AMP kinase is activated, your ability to convert dietary calories into chemical energy becomes super-efficient.

Properly restricting calories without malnutrition is one way to activate this enzyme of life. The other way to activate this enzyme of life is to consume high levels of polyphenols, such as those ingested by drinking three glasses of red wine per day as Luigi Cornaro did. Cornaro was using both dietary approaches simultaneously to extend his life. Another way to look at this is that the fewer polyphenols you consume (the more white carbohydrates you eat) and the more calories you consume, the faster you age. The Mediterranean Zone allows you to replicate Luigi's dual program of calorie restriction and high levels of polyphenols without needing to down three glasses of red wine a day on a highly restrictive diet.

One of the reasons people can't maintain calorie-restricted diets is that they are always fatigued. Consuming adequate levels of polyphenols, as found in the Mediterranean Zone, presents a solution to this problem. By activating the enzyme of life (AMP kinase) with adequate levels of polyphenols, your body is able to maintain high levels of chemical energy even in the presence of significant calorie restriction. As a result, you won't experience fatigue or hunger.

It is known that adherence to the traditional Mediterranean diet appears to be related to increased longevity. But is there any data that a specific group of nutrients in the traditional Mediterranean diet might be responsible for this increase in longevity?

Three such studies published in 2013 indicate that increased polyphenol intake may be the answer. The first two were epidemiology studies from Harvard Medical School. The first indicated that increased consumption of nuts (about 1 ounce per day) provided up to a 20 percent decrease in overall mortality. The other study indicated that consuming increased levels of berries generated up to a 32 percent reduction in heart attacks in women. The third study, in the *Journal of Nutrition*, demonstrated that the higher the levels of polyphenols absorbed (as measured by the polyphenol metabolites in the urine) by elderly subjects in Italy, the longer they were likely to live. How much longer? About 30 percent longer. Luigi Cornaro would be proud.

Today we spend billions of research dollars looking for new and expensive treatments for heart disease and cancer in order to live longer. However, the improvements in the death rates from these diseases are now becoming more limited as competing risks (such as Alzheimer's) are increasing. We are living longer, but maybe not better. In fact, there is also evidence that the improvement in the functional health status of elderly Americans halted more than a decade ago and that the length of our healthy lifespan (longevity minus years of disability) may actually be decreasing.

What we should be focusing on is how to delay aging—having a body and mind that are years younger than our actual chronological age, so we can be healthier and live a greater number of disability-free years. We don't have to spend billions of research dollars because the answer may lie with simply following the Mediterranean Zone and its recommendation to consume at least 1 gram of polyphenols and 2.5 grams of omega-3 fatty acids per day. In addition, consuming the types of meals shown in Chapter 5, you are restricting calories without hunger or fatigue when you follow the Mediterranean Zone. Combine them both and you live that longer and better life we all seek.

PART III

The Industrialization of Food

11

The Industrialization of Food and the Rise of Diet-Induced Inflammation

How did this epidemic of dietary-induced cellular inflammation begin in the first place? As with any tragedy, there is usually a good story behind it. The industrialization of the American diet essentially begins in the latter part of the nineteenth century when John Kellogg was the chief medical officer of a sanitarium operated by the Seventh-day Adventist Church in Battle Creek, Michigan. He was concerned about the lack of healthy gut function in his patients. (Perhaps *obsessed* might be a better word.) Kellogg was convinced the then-standard American breakfast of lard and bacon was killing people by clogging their colons. To test his theory that a healthy life begins with a healthy colon (including a lot of enemas), he starting experimenting by feeding his patients ready-to-eat breakfast cereals devoid of fat (and taste). His patients tolerated the stuff only because they were getting better. In 1904, C. W. Post, who had been a patient at the sanitarium, began production on a cereal similar to Kellogg's, but with a significant difference: He added extra sugar to make the bark-like material more palatable. The sugar he chose was grape sugar, chemically known as maltose, which consists of two glucose molecules linked together (basically a super sugar), and he named his new product Grape-Nuts. With that product, Post Cereals was born. What C. W. Post didn't realize was that maltose would rapidly break down to glucose, quickly increasing insulin levels and leading to constant hunger. I personally found this out as a young athlete who routinely consumed about six large bowls of Grape-Nuts every day. This may explain my lack of progress as a basketball player.

Grape-Nuts has been a wildly successful product for Post Foods. While John Kellogg, a nutritional purist, maintained that his cereal recipes needed no extra sugar, his brother, Will, was not so rigid. He figured that all that was needed for the family business to really succeed was to add sugar to the God-awful-tasting kitchen creations made by the company he and his brother had formed in 1897 to make unsweetened corn flakes and other equally unappealing products. His brother had no interest in compromising his dietary principles, so Will Kellogg formed his own new company in 1906 that eventually became the Kellogg Company. His older brother no longer spoke to him, but his new venture launched the cereal wars to win over the hearts and minds of Americans that continue to this day.

By 1916 James L. Kraft learned how to make processed cheese in days instead of months. He accomplished this by replacing traditional microbes with sodium phosphate and then pasteurizing the resulting product so it could last for years at room temperature in cans.

And we cannot forget about Milton Hershey, a pioneer in the polyphenol business—or at least the chocolate polyphenol business. He believed if he added even more milk and more sugar to chocolate he could make products that were cheaper than existing European chocolates made by companies such as Nestlé, and in the process everyone in America could afford to buy lots of his products. He was right, and the mass candy-bar business was born.

After the end of World War II the industrialization of food accelerated as companies such as General Mills, General Foods, and of course Kraft Foods started to mix science and engineering to make foods cheaper and more convenient. At the same time Big Food did a remarkable job of reducing the cost of food by stripping out the key components of unprocessed foods that reduced the shelf life (omega-3 fatty acids and polyphenols) and replacing them with much cheaper omega-6 fatty acids (and their chemically modified cousins, trans fats) and refined carbohydrates.

There were benefits to this new industrialization. The longer shelf life meant the possibility of globalizing their processed food production because spoilage was no longer a major issue. In addition, far fewer individuals were needed to actually produce enough food to feed a growing population. In the process, it started the largest mass migration in history, allowing hundreds of millions of people to move from rural areas to urban centers (especially in China) where more and more lucrative employment opportunities were possible. This migration from rural to urban areas still continues today as more than 50 percent of all people in the world now live in urban areas. In the United States, the percentage is more than 80 percent, as most of our population lives in urban and suburban areas. Since the percentage of urban dwellers is likely only to increase in the future, this means billions of individuals will be dependent on an industrialized global agribusiness industry for their daily food.

There are always some unintended health consequences of the industrialization and globalization of processed food. Not all crops are ideally suited for aggressive industrialization. The ones that were most suitable were wheat, corn, and soybeans. From wheat and corn come refined carbohydrates that rapidly enter the blood as glucose. From corn and soybeans come refined oils rich in omega-6 fatty acids. Through a combination of industrialization and farm subsidies, both refined carbohydrates high in glucose and oils rich in omega-6 fatty acids quickly became the cheapest sources of calories in the world. That made them the foundation of processed foods.

Unfortunately, this combination of food ingredients proved to be a deadly one. When high levels of insulin (responding to the rapid rise in blood glucose from refined carbohydrates) interacts with omega-6 fatty acids from soy, corn, and other vegetable and seed oils used to make the refined carbohydrates taste better, they accelerate the formation of arachidonic acid (AA) and, hence, set the stage for increased cellular inflammation.

Although refined carbohydrates such as white flour are the foundation for many processed foods, they taste like cardboard. Here the processed food industry learned to create a combination of ingredients that made their products so hard to resist for so many people: sugar, fat, and salt.

Humans have an innate desire for sugar. It is an ancient signal that indicated a food is probably safe to eat. We also know that the taste of sugar means that quick energy is coming our way to alleviate low blood sugar levels. Unfortunately, we now also know that sugar is potentially addictive. This realization comes from animal studies that indicate sugar may be more addictive than cocaine. One such animal study with mice has suggested the true potential severity of our sugar addiction. The mice were fitted with a backpack that injected them with cocaine after they had learned to press a lever a certain number of times. They quickly figured out the reward cycle and were seen in the throes of a full-on cocaine addiction. The researchers then placed super-sweetened sugar water (water saturatated with table sugar plus some extra artificial sweetener to make it a super-sugar) in the cages of cocaine-addicted mice. Within three days, the cocaine-addicted mice switched their allegiance from cocaine to the super-sweetened sugar water. Why the rapid conversion? Because both cocaine and glucose activate the same reward mechanisms used by dopamine in the brain. Since the super-sweetened sugar water has fewer side effects than the cocaine, the switchover wasn't a difficult choice to make.

Anytime you add sugar to a food product, such as tomato sauce or a breakfast cereal, people eat more of that product. This is why it is such an important ingredient in processed foods. However, there is a "bliss point" for sugar. Beyond a certain level in any food product the sugar level becomes *too* sweet and adding too much can create a "yuck" response. In other words, there is a zone (not to be confused with *the Zone you want to reach for maximum health and longevity*) and maintaining that range of sugar is the key to the appeal of processed foods.

Although we have identified taste receptors for sugar, no taste receptors for fat have been identified to date. Nonetheless, the processed food industry knows that there seems to be no bliss point for fat, especially if it is hidden from view (such as inside the crust of a Domino's pizza). Add a little sugar to that fat, and you have the formula for unlimited consumption. This is why fried dough without sugar isn't a popular item at the county fair, but if it is dusted with some sugar, you and your kids will be eating it all day long.

In the 1980s when fat was the "evil one," the only way to make fat-free processed foods palatable was to increase their sugar content, and just to be on the safe side, add some extra salt. Although the mechanism of how salt enhances taste is still debated, there is no question that adding it to any processed food makes the food more desirable to the consumer. That's because the hormonal reward networks in the brain activated by sugar, fat, and salt are essentially the same. So whenever one of three ingredients (sugar, fat, or salt) was out of fashion, increasing the levels of other two could compensate for its absence so that processed food would still have its addictive allure.

The globalization of food and the increasing use of processed foods are generating diet-induced inflammation on a global level. The rise of diabetes represents the best example of this rapid global spread of diet-induced inflammation. In Mexico, diabetes has increased 700 percent in the past twenty years. China now has more than 100 million diabetics (America has "only" 25 million), and there are more than 250 million diabetics worldwide. As I said previously, as the epidemic of diabetes increases, the stage is set for an equally rapid coming worldwide explosion of Alzheimer's.

12

Chasing the Wrong
Food Villains

It has become very trendy to try to assign the blame of our growing health-care crisis to a single food ingredient. I wish diet-induced inflammation were that simple. There is, at least, one artificial food ingredient that everyone agrees should be removed from every diet: trans fatty acids.

Recently the FDA announced a potential ban on trans fatty acids. Well, not exactly, since the FDA has never approved of them as food additives in the first place. They just kind of happened. First developed by Procter & Gamble (America's premier soap company) in the early 1900s, trans fatty acids quickly became a cheaper alternative to lard and butter as a source of fat with the introduction of Crisco into the American diet. Fortunately, Crisco tasted terrible. It was only with the advent of World War II and the rationing of butter that gave trans fatty acids their real push in the American diet in the form of margarine. Since trans fats are made from vegetable oils rich in omega-6 fatty acids, good marketing (led by the American Heart Association) convinced most Americans that they were "healthier" because they contained less saturated fat as well as being less expensive than butter.

American consumers continued to embrace shortening and margarine as alternatives to butter until initial research in the late 1980s indicated maybe these miracle fats weren't such a health bargain after all as evidence began mounting that trans fats seemed to be associated with increasing the risk of heart disease instead of lowering it.

However, by this time the processed food industry had learned to love trans fats. They were needed for manufactured products with an extended shelf life that could stand up to long-distance transport and an even longer life on the supermarket shelves without going rancid. The traditional method of adding saturated fats (such as lard) was no longer economical, but making lard-like fats from liquid vegetable oils was a way out of their shelf-life problem. Vegetable oils are a cheap source of calories, and the process to transform them into stable trans fats needed for extended shelf life is equally inexpensive.

Today it is still not certain why trans fats are so bad for us at the molecular level. We do know that the more trans fatty acids you consume, the more likely you are to develop heart disease. The usual suspects as to why they increase heart disease, such as lowering good cholesterol and increasing bad cholesterol (which trans fats do), are unlikely to explain why trans fatty acids also increase cellular inflammation. One theory is that trans fatty acids inhibit the formation of beneficial long-chain omega-3 fatty acids by interfering with key enzymes in their production. Another theory is that trans fatty acids make cell membranes more rigid, making it more difficult for hormones to transmit their signals to the interior of the cell. While the medical community agrees that trans fatty acids are detrimental to health, there are still a lot of remaining nagging questions about the actual mechanism of trans fats and how to explain their association with increased heart disease.

The Lyon Diet Heart Study, discussed earlier, demonstrated the difficulty in understanding the extent mechanism of trans fatty acids. In that study, subjects in the experimental group who were consuming margarine rich in trans fatty acids had 70 percent fewer heart attacks than the group consuming high amounts of omega-6 fatty acids. This remains, to my knowledge, the only long-term intervention study with trans fatty acids, and it generated just the opposite results than expected. This is not to say that trans fats were good, only that they were less harmful than the omega-6 fats that the control group was consuming. In fact, recent studies looking at all the data in cardiovascular patients who had replaced saturated fats with only omega-6 fats came to the conclusion that increasing the levels of omega-6 fatty acids seems to increase cardiovascular mortality.

Regardless of the questions on the mode of action of trans fatty acids posed by the results of the Lyon Diet Heart Study, the public outcry against trans fatty acids required the processed food industry to quickly look for a substitute that was almost as cheap as trans fatty acids. They found the solution in interesterified fats, a man-made fat created by combining totally hydrogenated vegetable oils with unsaturated vegetable oils. These interesterified fats contain no trans fatty acids, but studies have indicated this new type of fat may have the unintended consequence of causing increased insulin resistance. This is another case of "shoot, ready, aim" by the processed food industry.

There is no clear molecular mechanism to explain the association of trans fatty acids or potentially interesterified fats with chronic disease. Keep in mind trans fatty acids were developed as a replacement for saturated fats because of the crusade started by the American Heart Association to remove saturated fats from the American diet, as they were perceived to be the "real" cause of heart disease. (Sidebar: McDonald's used to fry its French fries in beef tallow, which is similar to lard. But after the publicity campaign started by Nebraska businessman Phil Sokolof generated such negative publicity, they replaced lard and beef tallow with trans fats.) However, in 2010 Harvard did another observational study indicating that there seemed to be no association of saturated fats with heart disease. This means the push by the American Heart Association for using omega-6 acids to replace saturated fats was probably never justified in the first place.

But what about the newest dietary "villains," which, unlike trans fats, are natural food ingredients that have been in the human diet for thousands of years? These include carbohydrates, fructose, milk, and gluten. Or the new dietary "hero," saturated fat? Unlike the scientific consensus on the negative effects of industrialized trans fatty acids (whatever the molecular reason), there remains great controversy relative to the role these food ingredients have in our current health-care crisis.

As I mentioned in the opening chapter, there is no magic bullet in nutrition, nor is there any single evil villain. Nutrition is far too complex to operate like that. This is why you have to search for a more comprehensive view to be consistent with all the data.

So let's look at these new dietary villains or heroes that are so popular in media headlines to see how strong the evidence is for each. In the process, I will also try to relate each to the real villain of our crumbling health, which is increased cellular inflammation.

Villain #1: Carbohydrates

The mantra of the Atkins diet is that carbohydrates increase insulin, and excess insulin makes you fat. Simply remove carbohydrates from your diet and replace them with fat. In fact, replace them with lots of saturated fats, such as bacon and heavily marbled porterhouse steaks. I totally agree with the problem of elevated insulin levels but not the proposed solution of the Atkins diet. It is true that carbohydrates (primarily glucose, since fructose has very little effect on insulin) do cause a transitory increase in insulin levels. But if you don't suffer from insulin resistance, then your insulin levels return to their normal levels quickly. The problem begins when insulin levels stay elevated all the time. Scientifically, this is called hyperinsulinemia, and it is caused by insulin resistance disrupting the signals between the insulin at the surface of the cell and the message it is trying to transmit to the interior of the cell. Insulin resistance is one of the first metabolic consequences of increased cellular inflammation. The cause of cellular inflammation is not carbohydrates *per se,* but the deadly *combination* of elevated insulin and omega-6 fatty acids.

Eventually you have to do clinical studies to back up your theories. I published one such study in the *American Journal of Clinical Nutrition* in 2006 comparing the Zone Diet to the Atkins diet. In this study, twenty obese individuals had all their meals prepared for them in a metabolic kitchen at Arizona State University. For six weeks half of the subjects were on the Zone Diet, the other half followed the Atkins diet. Each group ate the same number of daily calories for six weeks using prepared meals, following the guidelines for each respective diet program. During that time those subjects on the Zone Diet lost more weight, lost more fat, had more endurance activity, and were happier (using a standard psychological test) than those following the Atkins diet in this highly controlled study. More ominously, the Atkins diet doubled the levels of cellular inflammation in only six weeks. A more recent study from Harvard Medical School indicated that subjects on the Atkins diet (compared to subjects who ate the same number of calories but with more carbohydrates and less fat) had higher levels of cortisol, a stress hormone known for its deleterious effect on increasing fat accumulation, specifically abdominal fat, and lower levels of thyroid hormone, which causes fatigue and depression.

On a low-carbohydrate diet, you also have the problem of brain fog. Unlike other organs in the body, the brain can't use fat for energy. Because the brain is 60 percent fat, this would lead to the very undesirable situation of the brain cannibalizing itself to make energy. That's why the brain needs a constant supply of glucose in the blood for its energy needs. If glucose is not present in sufficient levels in your diet, then the body secretes more of the stress hormone cortisol to break down muscle mass to make more glucose. This is known as neo-glucogenesis. That's exactly what the Harvard research demonstrated. Since the brain needs about 130 grams of glucose per day, it makes sense to eat approximately that amount of carbohydrate each day. The rest of your body can easily live off stored fat, but the brain can't.

Robert Atkins was moving in the right direction by trying to reduce carbohydrates, but he took a major step backward by increasing saturated fats (which can increase cellular inflammation by binding to toll-like receptors) and forcing the body into abnormal hormonal responses (increased cortisol and decreased thyroid) by restricting carbohydrates too much.

Villain #2: Fructose

The three major carbohydrates you consume are glucose (coming from grains and starches), fructose (coming from fruits and vegetables), and galactose (coming from dairy products). Rather than taking all three carbohydrates out of the diet to get a low-carb diet such as Atkins, maybe only one of the three was the problem. This idea came from a short letter to the *American Journal of Clinical Nutrition* in 2004 hypothesizing an association between the increased use of high-fructose corn syrup and increased obesity. Unfortunately, the authors of the letter neglected to mention that the total fructose consumption in America hadn't changed much because any increase in high-fructose corn syrup was matched by a corresponding decrease in refined table sugar consumption. Sucrose (table sugar) has nearly the same ratio of fructose to glucose (about equal proportions of each) as high-fructose corn syrup does.

Another important fact that the short letter sent to the *American Journal of Clinical Nutrition* failed to mention is that the intake of high-fructose corn syrup had already been in steady decline since 1999 with no effect on obesity statistics. In reality, the most rapid increase of any food ingredient in the past forty years has been the consumption of grains rich in glucose and omega-6 fatty acids, not fructose. This increase in glucose consumption means an increase in insulin levels, which, when combined with excess omega-6 fatty acids, translates into increased cellular inflammation.

Fructose, on the other hand, has very little effect on insulin levels. It is true the body metabolizes fructose differently than glucose. Since both fructose and glucose are highly reactive, the body works very hard to avoid letting either sugar stay in the blood too long. Fructose has very little impact on insulin levels because it goes directly to the liver to be slowly converted into glucose, lactic acid, and fat. Glucose, on the other hand, is driven by insulin into the liver and muscle cells (for conversion and long-term storage as glycogen) or into fat cells (for conversion to glycerol to aid the storage of fatty acids as triglycerides for long-term storage). As long as you don't have insulin resistance, this process works very effectively for controlling the blood levels of both sugars. Although most fructose is converted slowly to glucose in the liver, the fat that is produced in the liver from fructose is repackaged into LDL lipoproteins to deliver fat to other tissues in the body for conversion energy. (Fat is high-octane fuel that allows you to make far more ATP per gram than per gram of carbohydrate.) As long as you don't oversupply the body with fructose, then this is fine. Of course, if you force-feed the body with excess fructose (similar to force-feeding a duck grains in order to make foie gras—which literally translates as fatty liver) you might create some problems. Fruits are rich in fructose, whereas vegetables are far less so; if you eat a lot of vegetables and limited amounts of fruit, it is impossible to overwhelm the liver with fructose. Furthermore, in experiments where the levels of fructose and glucose are held constant, there was absolutely no difference between the two different types of simple sugars on obesity or metabolism.

It is true that fructose is slightly more reactive than glucose, thereby potentially causing higher levels of free radical formation. This is where polyphenols come in. As the most powerful anti-oxidants known, they keep any potential excess free radicals coming from fructose (as well as glucose) metabolism under strict control. Studies have shown that when rats are fed a high-fructose diet and supplemented with polyphenols, all the metabolic abnormalities induced by the high-fructose feeding disappear. This is one of the reasons an apple a day keeps the doctor away. The beneficial effects of the apple polyphenols outweigh the possible negative levels of fructose in an apple. Of course, two servings of broccoli a day do an even better job than an apple at keeping the doctor away. That's because there's less fructose in the broccoli than the apple. Although grains and starches are free of fructose, they are composed of 100 percent glucose. This means they will dramatically increase insulin levels (whereas fructose will not) and generate lots of free radicals in the process (glucose is also very reactive especially in the blood). You need lots of dietary polyphenols to keep those free radicals coming from both glucose and fructose under control. So simply eat a lot of vegetables, limited amounts of fruits, and forget the grains and starches.

Fructose is not the problem because you consume at least an equal amount of glucose with it. In fact, the glucose-to-fructose ratio in the American diet is about five to one (and has remained so for the past ninety years). The most likely suspect in our obesity epidemic may be increased glucose, not fructose, consumption. The real problem is when you consume too much glucose in the presence of excess omega-6 fatty acids. That's how you develop cellular inflammation.

Villain #3: Dairy

The third source of carbohydrates for most people is galactose, found primarily in milk and dairy products. The gut breaks down the lactose found in both mother's milk and cow's milk to the simple carbohydrate fragments glucose and galactose. Unlike glucose, the body has little need for galactose, but it can metabolize it through a separate pathway so it doesn't build up in the body. The problem comes when the body loses the ability to break down lactose in the gut. Since lactose can't be absorbed, it moves on to the colon. The 100 trillion bacteria living there love lactose, and ferment it, resulting in bloating (caused by gases released during fermentation), flatulence, diarrhea, nausea, and vomiting. About 70 percent of adult Europeans (and nearly 100 percent in northern European countries, such as Germany, Denmark, and other Scandinavian countries) still retain the ability to make the enzyme that breaks down lactose into glucose and galactose, so these genetically lucky people don't have any problems consuming milk or dairy products. However, it is estimated that about 50 percent of the adult Mediterranean population (and 65 percent of the global population) is not so lucky. Their inability to digest lactose led to some of the first uses of biotechnology about eight thousand years ago.

One way to reduce lactose is to make cheese from the milk. The cheese-making process separates the primary milk protein (casein) from other milk proteins (such as whey) by adding acid to the milk. As the pH of the milk is lowered, the casein forms clumps (curds), and the whey and lactose stay in the solution. Remember the nursery rhyme of Little Miss Muffett eating her curds and whey? That was biotechnology in action. The harder the cheese (such as Parmesan), the less lactose it contains. Another way to reduce lactose is to add bacteria to milk. The added bacteria ferment the lactose into lactic acid. This is how you make yogurt. For the 50 percent of adult Europeans in the Mediterranean regions who still can't digest lactose, the development of cheese (especially Parmesan) and yogurt provided a way out of their genetic dilemma. This is why cheese and yogurt are protein mainstays of the Mediterranean diet. Today, there is another high-tech alternative: the separation of lactose from milk to generate lactose-free milk.

One of the surprising facts about per capita milk consumption in the United States is that it has decreased by nearly 75 percent in the last forty years. Much of this was a consequence of the removal of milk subsidies by the Reagan administration. Farmers were producing too much milk, forcing the government to buy the excess and convert it into cheese for long-term storage. When the Department of Agriculture decided it was going stop buying milk, it also decided to increase its advertising budget to sell the oversupply of cheese. The Department of Agriculture's campaign to sell off its cheese overstock led to the rapid growth of cheese pizza as an integral part of the American diet (pizza does exist as a part of the Mediterranean diet, but in Italy pizza is primarily composed of vegetables over a very thin crust), followed by the multi-cheese pizza, followed by the multi-cheese pizza with extra cheese stuffed into the crust. In this continuing transformation, a food that used to be considered an appetizer or dessert to be eaten in small portions as part of the Mediterranean diet quickly became a major source of calories in the American diet. The American intake of cheese has increased by 300 percent in the past forty years, and I guarantee most of that increase was not coming from artisanal cheeses.

There remains the issue of a possible allergic reaction to milk protein. However, if you eat too much of any one type of protein (even tofu), there is the potential to develop an allergy to it. The usual sources of allergies are proteins in various food ingredients. The primary offenders are milk, eggs, peanuts (actually a legume), nuts, fish, shellfish, soy, and wheat. Of these "big eight," four of these foods (eggs, nuts, fish, and shellfish) were also around in Paleolithic times, so protein-based food allergies are not totally a consequence of the advent of agriculture.

Milk allergies are more common in young children (about 3 to 5 percent of children), but about 90 percent of children outgrow their allergy by age 3. If you are a part of the 0.5 percent of the adult population with an allergy to milk protein, the usual indications are increased mucus formation in the nasal passages and the throat, sneezing, a runny nose, hives, or swelling of the lips, mouth, or throat when you consume milk. However, this also means that 99.5 percent of the population has no problems with milk protein, assuming most of the lactose has been removed. The number of people with an allergy to milk proteins are surprisingly similar to those with an allergy to another common protein in the diet: gluten. Bottom line, if you don't have any apparent allergies to dairy protein, then feel free to add a little Parmesan cheese or yogurt to your Mediterranean Zone meals.

Before I let dairy products off the hook completely, I need to discuss the effect of dairy protein on insulin secretion. Protein, such as carbohydrate, can also stimulate insulin release. Dairy products are powerful stimulators of insulin secretion. On the other hand, eggs have the least insulin-stimulating ability, followed by beef and fish. If you are consuming excess omega-6 fatty acids, then combining that with dairy products can possibly stimulate arachidonic acid formation and increased cellular inflammation. The increased cellular inflammation may be a major contributor to potential allergies coming from dairy products.

Villain #4: Gluten

Proteins, such as bacteria, normally don't enter into the bloodstream, thanks to the second skin that lines the digestive system. The lining of the gut is normally a tight barrier that allows only highly digested dietary components (single sugars, fatty acids, and very small protein peptides) that will not trigger allergenic reactions to enter the body. Of course, all bets are off if you have a leaky gut. A leaky gut is just that: Your second skin no longer acts as an effective barrier to prevent larger molecules such as intact proteins or large protein fragments from entering the blood. If they enter the bloodstream, they will be recognized as alien and will start a powerful immune reaction to this protein just as if bacteria or toxins were starting to breach the same barrier and entering the bloodstream.

There are two types of people with gluten problems. The first group has celiac disease, which represents true gluten intolerance. Those with celiac disease represent less than 1 percent of the population. These people simply cannot tolerate any gluten in the diet. My wife has severe celiac disease, so I know the consequences. The second group consists of those individuals who are gluten sensitive. They have few distinct clinical markers to gluten but seem to feel better when they don't eat gluten-containing products.

It is possible that the current epidemic of gluten sensitivity (not celiac disease) may be an indication that we really have a leaky gut epidemic. The most likely suspect in generating leaky gut syndrome is cellular inflammation, not gluten. In other words, gluten doesn't cause inflammation; however, existing inflammation in the lining of the gut can cause sensitivity to gluten. In particular, leaky gut syndrome is mediated by a subgroup of inflammatory eicosanoids known as leukotrienes, which are derived from arachidonic acid (AA). As AA levels increase (and EPA levels decrease) in the cells that line the gut, the stage is set for a growing percentage of these people to develop leaky gut syndrome. They become far more susceptible to a wide variety of immunological insults from any antigen-producing chemical (foods or chemicals) entering the bloodstream that would be otherwise prevented from doing so by a healthy gut lining.

Recent books have put forward a number of hypotheses about the connections between wheat, obesity, and chronic disease. The question is: Are these hypotheses justified? One of these assertions is that the increase in wheat consumption correlates well with the obesity epidemic. As I have pointed out, simply consuming carbohydrates doesn't make you fat per se, but the constantly elevated insulin levels caused by insulin resistance generated by cellular inflammation will do a very effective job of packing on the pounds. To increase cellular inflammation, you need the combination of excess refined carbohydrates coupled with excess omega-6 fatty acids. And omega-6 fatty acid consumption has grown at an even faster rate than wheat consumption.

The second proposed reason for gluten sensitivity is that the starch in wheat is thought to break down differently than other carbohydrates and enter the bloodstream more rapidly as glucose. This isn't true. The starches in white potatoes and white rice enter the bloodstream as glucose even faster than those from wheat, but it's not carbohydrates per se that cause insulin resistance, but cellular inflammation that can be driven by the initial insulin surge when coupled with excess omega-6 fatty acids.

The third argument driving the wheat-is-evil movement is that the glycemic index of wheat is higher than table sugar. That's true because table sugar is half fructose, which has little effect on insulin secretion. However, it is not the glycemic index of a carbohydrate but the glycemic load of the total meal that is important in determining the amount of insulin that will be secreted. When you balance the glycemic load of a meal by adding adequate amounts of low-fat protein (as you do following the Mediterranean Zone), you don't get a massive rise in blood glucose levels that leads to elevated insulin levels.

Finally, it has been hypothesized that the metabolism of gluten proteins produce powerful narcotic-like protein fragments that make you addicted to wheat. It is true that when a seven-peptide fragment of wheat is incubated with nerve cells, it can induce opioid-like effects. However, protein fragments of that size do not pass into the blood, let alone enter the brain, if you have a healthy gut (and a healthy blood-brain barrier). Only peptides containing two or three amino acids can pass across a healthy gut lining. Peptides of that limited size are too small to cause any type of immunological reaction, much less act as addictive agents. Of course, all bets are off if you have a leaky gut in which much larger things (such as whole bacteria, microbial fragments, intact protein such as gluten, and so on) can enter the bloodstream and play havoc with our immune system.

What causes a leaky gut? It comes from increased cellular inflammation in the cells that make up the lining of the gut membrane. Following the Mediterranean Zone is an excellent way to start to heal a leaky gut if you are gluten sensitive. As your gut inflammation decreases, you might consider adding some grains back into your diet to see how the healing process is going. The only two grains I would suggest are slow-cooked oatmeal and barley because they are both rich in soluble fiber that slows down carbohydrate entry into the blood, lowering the glycemic response. However, I wouldn't go beyond those two sources of grains.

So why do people feel better when they go on a gluten-free diet? For the same reason that they feel better on the Zone Diet. You are removing high-glycemic load carbohydrates from your diet, making it more difficult to maintain arachidonic acid levels that ultimately cause a leaky gut. This improvement can be accelerated if you are reducing your intake of omega-6 fatty acids at the same time. For most Americans, the primary sources of gluten are bread, pasta, and pastries. Take these food items out of the diet, and you significantly lower the glycemic load and when that happens, you lose weight and feel better.

I firmly believe that cutting out all grains from the diet is an excellent idea. In fact, I was quoted in *Time* magazine in 1997 stating, "If all the bread left the face of the earth, we would have a much healthier planet." My quote was based on the importance of reducing the glycemic load of the diet, not the removal of gluten. I haven't changed my opinion. You won't starve to death if you replace those high-glycemic carbohydrates with lots of vegetables and limited amounts of fruits, which provides more anti-inflammatory polyphenols with far fewer carbohydrates.

There is a grain of nutritional truth in all of these new dietary villains. However, they don't cause inflammation; they are secondary consequences of an inflamed gut caused by pre-existing cellular inflammation. That's why they are not a panacea for addressing chronic disease. Your primary "drug" to reduce diet-induced inflammation is following the Mediterranean Zone. Only once you have mastered that dietary intervention as indicated by reaching the clinical markers that define the Zone, then think about reducing (not totally eliminating) these new dietary "villains." If you are already in the Zone, then you probably won't see much difference as you reduce their levels because they are already minor food ingredients in the Mediterranean Zone.

Villain #4: Saturated Fat

Although there is no epidemiological link between saturated fat and heart disease, that doesn't mean saturated fat is good for you. While saturated fat is not nearly as inflammatory as omega-6 fatty acids, it can induce cellular inflammation by interacting with one of the toll-like receptors on the surface of every cell in the body. Saturated fats can fool this receptor into thinking the cell is under microbial attack. Intervention studies have continuously demonstrated that saturated fats are more inflammatory than monounsaturated fats. If you want to add fat to your diet, then add extra-virgin olive oil instead of vegetable oils such as safflower, corn, or soybean.

The real villain we should be seeking to control in our battle against obesity and its associated diseases is diet-induced inflammation. The trouble with pointing the finger at a single dietary food ingredient as a "villain" is that you are overlooking the complex relationships in nutrition, which makes it more likely that you will continue to suffer the health consequences of increased cellular inflammation.

PART IV

The Future of Medicine

13

Epigenetics:
Opening Pandora's Genetic Box

I n 2005 an article in the *New England Journal of Medicine* predicted that the potential lifespan of children born in the twenty-first century would be less than their parents'. The authors of the study further estimated that one out of every three children born after 2000 will likely develop diabetes. If this projection is valid, then by 2050 about one-third of adult Americans may have diabetes compared to the current 11 percent today. Since diabetes will most likely continue to develop at a much earlier age, this means a longer duration of the disease. As a consequence, many of those children born after 2000 who develop diabetes are also more likely to develop Alzheimer's. This may represent the breaking point for an already overwhelmed health-care system by 2050. So how did we get into this morass in which each generation seems to become fatter and sicker?

The answer may lie in the strange new science of trans-generational epigenetics in which diet-induced inflammation is transmitted and amplified from one generation to the next.

Epigenetics refers to changes in gene function that do not involve direct changes (such as mutations) in the DNA sequence of our genetic code. Like a molecular light switch, epigenetics allows genes to be modified sometimes temporarily, sometimes permanently by environmental factors such as diet. Epigenetics also explains how the future expression of the genes of an unborn child can be altered by the diet of his parents and possibly his grandparents to have exaggerated inflammatory responses throughout the rest of his life. Our growing obesity epidemic in the young and the earlier development of diabetes may be indications that the genes of our children are being reprogrammed with potentially very adverse future health consequences. But to truly understand the importance of epigenetics, we have to go back in time to when we thought that genetics was much simpler to understand.

In 2000 it was announced with great fanfare that the human genetic code had been finally sequenced. Genetics was going to usher in a new era of personalized medicine. There was new potential hope for seeing into the future to determine what diseases were lurking in your genome and taking steps to prevent them, or at least find the right drug to treat them more effectively when they did arise. After the initial hype faded, it turns out there were still a lot of unanswered questions about our genes. It didn't appear that the human genome was all that different from that of a chimpanzee. In fact, many plants (such as wheat and corn) had a far greater number of genes than we do. Additionally, there seemed to be a lot of "junk" DNA (actually 98 percent of the DNA) in the human gene that didn't appear to do anything useful such as make proteins. After all, that's what twenty-five thousand "real" genes in human DNA do.

Now we know genetics is a lot more complicated than we imagined. The number of human genes aren't all that much greater in number or uniquely different from other species; however, it does appear that our genes can be turned on and off with far greater precision and speed than in other animals (or plants). Much of that increased sophisticated gene activity is due to the presence of microRNA fragments found within all that "junk" DNA. Finally, many of the gene transcription factors that turn on or off selected gene sequences of your DNA (such as those that control the production of inflammatory proteins or anti-oxidant proteins) seem to be affected by key nutrients such as omega-3 fatty acids and polyphenols.

Your DNA doesn't exist in an isolated form. Proteins called histones surround the DNA. If these histones are tightly wrapped around the DNA, it can't be replicated. If the histones are looser, then DNA can be replicated. What controls the opening and closing of histones are chemical modifications along their surface. In addition, there can also be transitory chemical modifications of the DNA itself. If a section of the DNA is chemically altered, then it becomes silent and can't be replicated. These epigenetic chemical modifications don't change the actual gene structure, but they do determine whether or not that section of the DNA can make proteins based on the code of the DNA. Finally there is the role of microRNAs, which come from all that "junk" DNA. Although these microRNA fragments can't be used as a template to make proteins coded by the genes, they can inhibit the synthesis of potential proteins by interfering with the processing necessary for the synthesis of that particular protein. It is best to think of your DNA as the hardware in your genes, and epigenetics and gene transcription factors as its software.

The complexity of epigenetics in humans gives us a tremendous flexibility to live in a wide number of climates, from the Arctic to the Amazon. It represents a very elegant control system that allows slight genetic adjustments to changes in dietary, environmental, and stress levels. But it also makes our genes prone to being hijacked by an inflammatory diet.

The one time in your life that your environment has the greatest effect on your future gene expression via epigenetics is while you are in the womb. The mother's diet establishes many of these epigenetic chemical marks on the fetal DNA to prepare it for the world that awaits it after birth. If there is a mismatch of the epigenetic programming taking place in the womb and the environment the newborn child actually experiences, there will be trouble ahead, usually in the form of the increased likelihood of obesity, diabetes, and heart disease.

The first indication that dietary changes could affect future populations came during World War II. As the German troops were retreating from the Netherlands in the winter of 1944, they took all available food with them, creating a severe famine for the Dutch citizens left behind. It was estimated that the average calorie intake per person during what was known as the Dutch Famine was about 600 calories per day. After the war, both prosperity and food quickly returned to the Netherlands and all seemed well. Then in 1999 researchers began studying the population records of the women who were in their last trimester of pregnancy during the Dutch Famine. Their children were more obese and had higher rates of diabetes and heart disease compared to children who were born either before or after the Dutch Famine. It became apparent that the calorie restriction experienced by their mothers more than fifty years earlier had resulted in negative health consequences for their children in the womb. Scientists call this fetal programming. It is especially powerful in the last trimester of pregnancy when the mother's diet greatly influences the epigenetic changes to the fetal DNA to prepare them for what their new environment will be outside the womb. During the Dutch Famine there was a complete mismatch of the mother's diet during their pregnancy relative to what the dietary environment their child would experience after their birth. The result was these children had an altered metabolism—one that was suited to famine conditions, rather than abundance. This epigenetic mismatch resulted in increased incidence of obesity, diabetes, and heart disease. The fact that all these conditions (obesity, diabetes, and heart disease) are linked by increased diet-induced inflammation suggests that some of those epigenetic changes taking place during the Dutch Famine may also have turned on selected genes that resulted in enhanced diet-induced inflammation once adequate food was available. This is because the fetus was programmed in the womb for highly restricted calorie intake conditions, which was totally mismatched for abundance of calories available after the birth.

At the same time as the Dutch Famine, similar famine conditions were occurring in Leningrad. However, after the war there was not any greatly increased food supplies in Russia. As a result, there was no increase in obesity, diabetes, or heart disease in their children as they became adults. The fetal programming that took place in the wombs of Russian mothers during these famine conditions was ideally matched to the dietary environment their children were born into.

During the first two years of life you are very susceptible to laying down diet-induced epigenetic marks on your DNA. This may be one of the reasons breast-fed children seem to have both better health and higher IQs compared to those children raised on infant formulas. If you look at the composition of virtually every infant formula (another product of the industrialization of food), you will see they are primarily composed of sugar and omega-6 fatty acids. This is a sure-fire prescription for increased diet-induced inflammation primed to do even more epigenetic mischief.

These epigenetic marks established in fetal programming or early postnatal eating patterns can last a lifetime. Furthermore, they can be transmitted and even amplified from one generation to the next, depending on the dietary environment in which the next generation of parents consumes. If epigenetic changes can increase inflammation, then is it possible that diet-induced inflammation can induce epigenetic changes? Unfortunately, the answer may be yes.

Animal models demonstrate all too clearly the genetic consequences of a continuing inflammatory diet on future generations. In one very disturbing study published in 2009, researchers took genetically identical mice and split them into two colonies. The diets of the mice were identical in terms of calories, protein, carbohydrate, and total fat. The only difference was that in one group the fat content was richer in omega-6 fatty acids and poorer in omega-3 fatty acids. This was a seemingly minor change, especially since both sets of mice were on low-fat diets. These colonies were maintained under these same dietary conditions for three generations. The weight gain wasn't instantaneous in the first generation of the mice getting higher omega-6 fatty acid intake, but by the third generation, those mice consuming the higher levels of omega-6 fatty acids were grossly obese compared to their genetically identical cousins. These changes were induced by cellular inflammation caused by the change to the proportion of omega-6 fatty acids to omega-3 fatty acids in their diet. In subsequent studies, the same researchers demonstrated that if you increase the levels of omega-6 fatty acids in the diet of the mice to the same levels in the current American diet, the faster the obesity develops.

More ominously, there were also significant metabolic changes being transmitted from one generation to the next. By the third generation of mice getting the higher levels of omega-6 fatty acids, there were significant indications of pre-diabetes, indicated by fatty deposits in the liver and early signs of heart disease, indicated by enlarged hearts.

So let's look at the rise in obesity in the American population during the time in which similar changes in the ratio of omega-6 to omega-3 fatty acids were also changing in the American diet.

1960: 13%
1980: 15%
1994: 23%
2000: 31%
2010: 36%

This nearly 300 percent increase in obesity in three generations suggests that Americans seem to be following the same trans-generational epigenetic trend as seen in the animal studies as a consequence of increased intake of omega-6 fatty acids and corresponding decrease in omega-3 fatty acids.

Unfortunately, the industrialization of food in the last three generations has become a powerful force in changing the epigenetic marks that control the genetic future of our children as well as ourselves. Perhaps not surprisingly, the fastest growing group of obese individuals in America is children born after the year 2000. The odds of them achieving a normal weight and having a healthy future were stacked against them before they ever left the womb.

This is also true of neurological outcomes. If you make mice deficient in omega-3 fatty acids for several generations, they become increasingly more anxious, less focused, and less intelligent compared to their genetically identical cousins who were getting adequate levels of omega-3 fatty acids during the fetal period and thereafter. No wonder ADHD, anxiety, and depression are becoming epidemic in America's children.

Epigenetic changes may become permanent if the environmental factors (such as an inflammatory diet) are maintained. The growth of the industrialization of the American food supply may be a driving force in an epigenetic shift in our genes that could be responsible for the epidemic rise of obesity, diabetes, and eventually Alzheimer's.

There is no easy way of out this genetic storm, because it takes about two to three generations to totally erase these epigenetic marks from DNA, and that's assuming you have removed the offending dietary causes in the first place. That's why following the Mediterranean Zone may be the best possible "drug" we have to cope with diet-induced epigenetic changes in ourselves, our children, and their future children. The Mediterranean Zone can hold back many of the epigenetic changes leading to increases to our inflammatory genes induced by prior fetal programming. For each succeeding generation following the Mediterranean Zone, there will be a continuing reduction in those epigenetic markers laid down generations earlier. Within three generations, those epigenetic changes induced by pro-inflammatory diets in the past should be erased completely. The dietary changes needed to follow the Mediterranean Zone are comparatively small compared to the future health benefits for generations to come.

14

Reclaiming Our Genetic Future

Nutrition is complex, and yet we seem to continually try to dumb it down in the media by using political-like slogans based on simplistic thinking that is often not supported by the facts. In the late twentieth century, saturated fat caused heart disease. Today, the recent campaigns against new single classes of nutrients (fructose, dairy, gluten) completely miss the point as to why the health of Americans is rapidly deteriorating. I wish it were possible to simply remove one food ingredient from the American diet and suddenly return our population to the land of milk and honey (oops, two of the "evil ones"), but it's not possible.

Nutrition is not like mathematics where you deal in certainties and elegant proofs. Nutrition is based on probabilities. There are some dietary statements that I think have different degrees of probability.

#1. There is a high probability that our diet can induce inflammation.

The 1982 Nobel Prize in Medicine was awarded for linking eicosanoids to inflammation. Depending on the fats you eat, you either make pro-inflammatory or anti-inflammatory eicosanoids. If those fats are rich in omega-6 fatty acids coupled with a diet consisting of high-glycemic load carbohydrates that increases insulin levels, then you will rapidly escalate diet-induced inflammation. On the other hand, a diet rich in omega-3 fatty acids and polyphenols coupled with low-glycemic load carbohydrates to prevent excess insulin levels will reduce diet-induced inflammation.

#2. There is a good probability that constantly elevated insulin, a consequence of insulin resistance, is caused by diet-induced inflammation.

The higher the glycemic load of a meal, the more insulin you produce. That's okay as long as insulin is doing its job correctly, because if you don't have insulin resistance, those elevated levels of insulin after a meal will quickly return to normal. However, all bets are off once you develop insulin resistance because the target cells (fat, liver, and muscle) dependent on insulin's ability to remove glucose and fat from the bloodstream become less efficient. Because of this disruption in insulin's action in targeted cells, the pancreas secretes more insulin to reduce the elevated levels of glucose and fats in the bloodstream. As a consequence, the levels of insulin in the blood will remain elevated all the time. If you also are consuming high levels of omega-6 fatty acids in your diet, then the combination of these two factors will increase the levels of arachidonic acid, which further increases cellular inflammation. The combination of these two dietary factors (elevated insulin and increased omega-6 fatty acids) speeds up the development of chronic disease and accelerates the aging process.

3. There is a reasonable probability that the lack of omega-3 fatty acids in the diet is making it difficult to control chronic cellular inflammation.

The resolution of inflammation is a totally distinct process from the initiation of inflammation. Without the consumption of adequate levels of both omega-3 fatty acids in the diet, the resolution phase of inflammation is weak, and this allows the inflammation to continue at chronic low levels in every organ in your body. Eventually, if there is enough organ damage, we call it chronic disease.

4. There is a reasonable probability that our increasingly pro-inflammatory diet is modifying gene expression to constantly fuel the inflammatory fires in every cell in the body.

Our diet is one of the primary environmental factors that control gene expression, especially inflammatory genes. The more inflammation you create by your diet, the more inflammatory genes are activated to continue to produce a continuing stream of inflammatory proteins that maintains chronic cellular inflammation. The end result is that you become fatter and sicker and accelerate the aging process. As long as we maintain our pro-inflammatory diets, epidemics of obesity and diabetes (and Alzheimer's) are all but assured in our future.

#5. Epigenetic changes induced by pro-inflammatory diets might be amplified and transmitted from one generation to the next, increasing the chances that obesity and the early development of chronic disease will become the new normal for generations to come.

This last possibility is truly frightening as our quest for cheaper and more convenient industrialized food may be causing genetic manipulations of the human genome for the worse.

Just as I believe that nutrition is more complex than we are told, I equally believe that the practice of medicine is not as complex as we think. In essence, if you control diet-induced inflammation in your body, you will lead a longer and healthier life. That's why I believe that the future practice of medicine should be composed of three distinct steps:

1. Individuals should focus their dietary efforts on getting as close to the Zone as possible. This is totally dependent on the individual because the clinical markers that define the Zone are controlled by the diet. I don't particularly feel strongly about what diet you follow as long as you can reach those markers that define the Zone. However, I believe that the Mediterranean Zone provides the easiest way to achieve those clinical markers with the least dietary stress on your part. This is especially true if you already have an existing chronic disease.
2. Diet is not going to totally replace drugs, but it does make drugs work better at lower concentrations. The closer you are to the Zone

(as defined by its clinical markers), the fewer drugs you will need to treat the remaining symptoms of chronic disease. Today we have it backward. We overmedicate patients with drugs in an attempt to overcome the effects of a pro-inflammatory diet that are the underlying causes of chronic disease. Ideally the cost of health care would be adjusted to reflect how closely a person was to the Zone. Those markers that define the Zone can also be used to define wellness, and in particular provide "evidence-based wellness" for the benefits of the diet. People would get significant reductions in the cost of their health care based on their ability to maintain their wellness.

3. We have to start making the financial incentives for physicians based on maintaining wellness as opposed to treating the symptoms of chronic disease. Maintenance of wellness is very different from the prevention of chronic disease. Wellness can be easily measured and compensated for success. This is sustainable health care. Paying for the treatment of symptoms with increasingly expensive drugs and procedures is not sustainable.

This may seem low-tech in comparison to today's high-tech medicine. However, I am certain that anything less than this three-step model of health care will be unsustainable in terms of future health-care costs. This plan does not require new breakthroughs in biotechnology but does require a new model of medicine that recognizes the power of diet as its primary "drug" and the need for the patient to be part of the solution. This is not new thinking, as it is essentially what Hippocrates proposed 2,500 years ago when he said, "Let food be your medicine, and let medicine be your food."

There is one country that is using this approach on a society-wide basis: Japan. Although the Japanese are the longest-lived population in the world with the greatest health span (total lifespan minus years of disability), they realize they too have growing problems with diabetes and Alzheimer's. Rather than throwing their hands up in despair, they took a rather unique approach to proactively treat what could one day become an epidemic that could destroy their entire economy. In 2007 all employers in Japan were given notice that they had five years to start reducing the number of their employees with metabolic syndrome (pre-diabetes) by 15 percent, and by 25 percent by the year 2015. If those requirements were not met, then the employers (not the employees) would be subject to a substantial tax to help pay for the projected future health-care expenses of their employees. Since Japan has a national health-care system that includes yearly checkups, the Japanese government had excellent insight into employee compliance. You can imagine the uproar if such a mandate were to be proposed in the United States or Europe. Yet the Japanese know this is a matter of national economic security, and they are willing to pay the price.

We either solve this problem of diet-induced inflammation in every socioeconomic sector of our society, or we will all fall together into a black hole of unimaginable health-care expenses in the future, as the incidence of obesity, diabetes, and Alzheimer's continues to increase. It may be through following the Mediterranean Zone as described in this book, or taxing the production of omega-6 fatty acids, or making vegetables essentially free by the use of vouchers (basically vegetable food stamps) for every segment of the population, or by following the Japanese example of taxation on employers to slow down the growth of diabetes and Alzheimer's. These may appear to be radical approaches, but each one provides the potential to help us retake control of our genetic future. We must realize that unless changes come quickly, we will all sink under the increasing weight of health-care expenses as diabetes and Alzheimer's continue to take their considerable health-care tolls. Furthermore, we need to have a solution that affects every economic sector of society, not just the economically elite that shop at Whole Foods. It will take significant capital to undertake such wide-scale changes, but unless those changes are implemented our future national security is at significant risk thanks to the extraordinary drain of future health-care costs on our financial resources.

Throughout this book, I have discussed how the industrialization of our food supply has set in motion an unprecedented change in the expression of inflammatory genes, presenting a very bleak health future for America. It will take the equivalent of a multi-generational "wartime effort" to reverse the epigenetic changes of the last fifty years. It remains to be seen whether or not we have the will to win that war to reclaim our genetic future, but I know this: A diet rich in omega-3 fatty acids and polyphenols and low in omega-6 fatty acids and refined carbohydrates is the most important part of medicine we have in reclaiming our health now and for future generations to come.

Appendix A

Continuing Support

The world of nutrition is constantly evolving, and we are now able to explore with growing scientific sophistication how our diet can affect the expression of our genes. To stay on top of that world, I can offer several resources. For the rapid acceleration of the science of nutrition, www.DrSears.com compiles breaking research news on nutrition and medicine on a daily basis. For advice and products that help support the Mediterranean Zone, I can recommend www.ZoneDiet.com. Likewise, one of the best markers of being in the Zone is the AA/EPA ratio. Used primarily in research studies, it is not a standard blood test, but it is available at the lowest possible cost at www.ZoneDiagnostics.com.

The Mediterranean Zone meals in this book are taken from the menu at the Saturnia Spa in Tuscany, Italy, considered one of the top spas in the world. The meals were developed by Dr. Daniela Morandi and Chef Claudio Colombo Severini. These Mediterranean Zone meals represent the foundation of Dr. Morandi's Nutritional Reset program at the Saturnia Spa.

Appendix B

The Science of Diet-Induced

Inflammation

Understanding the concept of the Zone means understanding the link between diet and inflammation. We often think of inflammation as harmful, whereas, in fact, it keeps us alive. Without a strong inflammatory response to fight off microbial invasion and help heal physical injuries, our future would be bleak. On the other hand, if those same inflammatory responses are not brought back to normal, then that resulting chronic low-level inflammation continues to attack our own tissue, leading to obesity, development of chronic disease, and acceleration of the aging process. In other words, you need a balance of inflammatory soldiers that can be called into action when needed and then returned to their barracks when the action is over.

The primary soldiers in your inflammation army are a group of hormones known as eicosanoids. Little is known by the medical profession about these hormones, even though the 1982 Nobel Prize in Medicine was awarded for understanding their role in the inflammatory process, and more than 125,000 scientific papers have been published about them.

My interest in eicosanoids began more than thirty years ago when I began to consider the impact of diet on eicosanoid formation and on inflammation. It is a complex story that I have told many times in my previous books, so here is a short summary.

Essential Fatty Acids

Essential fatty acids are fats that the human body cannot make and therefore must be supplied by the diet. The two key essential fatty acids that play a critical role in the body's inflammatory responses are the omega-6 fatty acid arachidonic acid (AA) and the omega-3 fatty acid eicosapentaenoic acid (EPA). It is the balance of AA and EPA that ultimately controls the degree of cellular inflammation in the body because these two fatty acids can be converted directly into the eicosanoids that ultimately control inflammation. The eicosanoids derived from omega-6 fatty acids (AA) are pro-inflammatory and accelerate inflammation; the eicosanoids derived from EPA are anti-inflammatory and are critical for the resolution of inflammation. The AA/EPA ratio in the blood provides a unique insight into the balance of these two fatty acids in every one of the 10 trillion cells in the body and describes how well you are able to maintain a healthy inflammatory response and, as a result, live a longer and better life. It was obvious to me decades ago as I was developing the Zone Diet that it could be used as a powerful "drug" to be taken at the right dose and at the right time to change the balance of these fatty acids and thus control the levels of inflammation in the body.

That part was easy to come up with. The more difficult process was to understand how the molecular pathways leading to these two fatty acids could be modified by the diet to optimize the ratio of AA and EPA to control inflammation. You need some AA to mount an inflammatory response to microbial invasions or to heal injuries; however, if the levels of AA are too high, the inflammatory response is constantly turned up, and the end result is that the body attacks itself. If there were too little EPA in the cell, there would be limited competition with AA for the enzymes (cyclo-oxygenase, or COX, and lipo-oxygenase, or LOX) that make inflammatory eicosanoids, thus making it impossible for the body to control inflammatory responses. On the other hand, if you have an excess of EPA in the cell, it might inhibit the inflammatory response too much, making it more difficult to repel microbial invaders.

In addition, from EPA (and the other long-chain omega-3 fatty acid docosahexaenoic acid, or DHA) comes a powerful group of anti-inflammatory eicosanoids known as resolvins that turn off the inflammatory response. It should be noted that the initiation of inflammation is totally different from the resolution of inflammation. *Anti-inflammation* can be thought of inhibition of the initiation phase of inflammation. *Pro-resolution* can be thought of as the acceleration of the termination of the inflammatory response. Both pathways (the initiation of inflammation and its resolution) have to be in balance to maintain inflammatory homeostasis. What was needed to achieve this was a dietary approach to maintain the AA/EPA ratio in a zone that is not too high, but not too low.

Obviously, one key to this challenge was reducing the intake of the omega-6 fatty acid precursor (linoleic acid) that is necessary for AA formation. For much of human history linoleic acid was a minor part of the human diet. That changed eighty years ago with the industrialization of vegetable oil processing that, virtually overnight, produced a flood of omega-6 rich vegetable oils (corn, soybean, sunflower, and safflower). These soon became the most inexpensive form of calories known on the face of the earth. As a result, the levels of linoleic acid in the human diet began to rise, first in America and then spreading worldwide through the globalization of food. That situation might have been tolerable, since there were two rate-limiting steps that control the flow of linoleic acid into AA.

Both of the key regulatory enzymes (delta-6 and delta-5 desaturase) that control the ultimate formation of AA are activated by insulin and are inhibited by the omega-3 fatty acids (EPA and DHA). Unfortunately, just as linoleic acid levels were beginning to increase in the human diet, so were the levels of refined carbohydrates that enter the bloodstream very quickly as glucose (thus increasing insulin) coupled with a dramatic drop in the dietary intake of omega-3 fatty acids.

The hormonal response to any rapidly rising blood glucose is an increased secretion of insulin. When high levels of linoleic acid combine with high levels of insulin, the result is increased AA formation. It's like adding a lighted match to a vat of gasoline. This is because insulin activates the key enzymes (delta-6 and delta-5 desaturases) needed to convert linoleic acid into AA. EPA and DHA can partially, but not totally, inhibit this metabolic consequence of the increased intakes of linoleic acid and refined carbohydrates. Thus the key to really controlling AA formation is not only the restriction of omega-6 fatty acids, but also restriction of high-glycemic carbohydrates as described in Chapter 3.

The more you control the intake of omega-6 fatty acids and high-glycemic carbohydrates, the less omega-3 fatty acids you need to keep your inflammatory responses in a healthy zone. Of course, the converse is also true. The more omega-6 fatty acids and high-glycemic carbohydrates you consume, the more omega-3 fatty acids you need to control excess AA formation. Even following a strict Mediterranean Zone dietary program, there is usually a need to supplement the diet with omega-3 fatty acids either from high fish consumption or supplementation with highly purified omega-3 fatty acids to help slow down the formation of AA as well as increase the rate of resolution of the inflammatory response.

Differences Between Omega-3 Fatty Acids

Just as omega-6 fatty acids drive inflammation, omega-3 fatty acids are the drivers of both anti-inflammation and pro-resolution. Well, some are. The most abundant omega-3 fatty acid is alpha-linolenic acid (ALA), which is found in high concentrations in certain seeds (flax and chia), leafy plants such as purslane, and nuts (walnuts being the highest). ALA has no anti-inflammatory properties unless it is transformed in the longer chain omega-3 fatty acids such as EPA and DHA. Unfortunately, this metabolic conversion is a very slow and inefficient process with only 1 and 5 percent of the ingested ALA becoming either DHA or EPA respectively. The oil found in fatty fish such as salmon, sardines, and anchovies, on the other hand, are rich in EPA and DHA. That is because they are at the end of the marine food chain that starts with algae, which make EPA and DHA readily. So if you want to gain the full anti-inflammatory and pro-resolution benefits of the Mediterranean Zone, plan to eat a lot of seafood. Until recently, fish was one of the main sources of protein in the Mediterranean diet before the high cost of fish and fears of toxins such as PCBs and mercury placed a real damper on this dietary practice. This is why purified omega-3 fatty acid supplements actually become a better choice than fish to enhance the benefits of the Mediterranean Zone.

EPA and DHA are quite different in their functions in the body. EPA is virtually identical to AA from a three-dimensional viewpoint. This is why it can inhibit the formation of pro-inflammatory eicosanoids by occupying the same binding site as AA on the key enzymes necessary for the further metabolism into eicosanoids. DHA has a very different three-dimensional structure, making it much more difficult to compete with AA for those key binding sites of the COX enzyme. (COX enzymes are responsible for making both pro-inflammatory and anti-inflammatory prostaglandins.)

This is why the AA/EPA ratio is such an excellent marker for determining the extent of cellular inflammation. The higher the AA/EPA ratio, the easier it is to make inflammatory eicosanoids. The lower the AA/EPA ratio, the more difficult it is. So from this standpoint, EPA is more anti-inflammatory than DHA, at least in the initiation phase of inflammation.

Although DHA has a hard time fitting into the COX enzyme, it is a different story for the LOX enzymes. Both EPA and DHA can inhibit the formation of LOX-derived inflammatory eicosanoids such as leukotriene derived from AA as well as forming powerful pro-resolution resolvins coming from the same LOX enzymes. You need a very low AA/EPA ratio (between 1.5 and 3) to get the maximum resolution of inflammation because you have to saturate the EPA-binding sites of the more abundant COX enzymes first so that enough of the remaining EPA gets pushed over to the LOX pathways to make even more resolvins. That's also why you always want a combination of EPA and DHA (with more EPA than DHA) to maximize the resolution of inflammation.

I believe the most appropriate AA/EPA ratio is that found in the longest-lived population in the world, the Japanese. The average AA/EPA ratio in the general Japanese population is about 1.5. For comparison, the average AA/EPA ratio in the American population is about 20. In older Italians (models for the Mediterranean diet), their AA/EPA was about 10 or about midway between the Americans and the Japanese. However, the AA/EPA ratio in the younger generation of Italians is rapidly increasing and is now equal to that of Americans, indicative of the impact of increasing consumption of both linoleic acid and refined carbohydrates through the globalization of industrialized foods as well as decreasing fish consumption.

There is also the constant need for DHA as well as EPA. DHA has such different structural properties compared to EPA, and it is more effective in creating greater fluidity in both membranes and lipoproteins. Fluidity is especially important in neural membranes that require a very flexible membrane surface to facilitate the transport of neurotransmitters to maintain nerve signaling. In addition, DHA tends to break up "lipid rafts" composed of saturated lipids and cholesterol in membranes. This often prevents the signaling of metastatic mediators needed for cancer growth.

You find EPA and DHA in every organ in the body to be relatively similar to their levels in the blood except in the brain, where the levels of EPA are negligible. This has led to a mistaken belief that EPA is not important for neural function, but nothing could be further from the truth. The brain is unique in that, unlike other organs in the body, the brain can't effectively make AA, EPA, or DHA from shorter chain omega-3 or omega-6 fatty acids. The vast majority of these longer-chain essential fatty acids have to be transported across the blood-brain barrier. The transport efficacy of all three is about the same, so the initial uptake of these fatty acids into the brain is roughly similar to their concentrations in the blood. However, once inside the brain, only the EPA is rapidly oxidized, whereas both AA and DHA are shuttled to long-term storage in the phospholipids of the neural membranes. Considering that EPA is critically important in every other organ as an anti-inflammatory compound, this seems to make no sense unless it is being oxidized into something that is even more important to the brain. I believe this is the case. The brain is extraordinarily sensitive to inflammatory damage. Therefore, it makes sense to oxidize the incoming EPA into resolvins, which act as constant anti-inflammatory sentinels to keep inflammation under control in the brain. However, resolvins have a very short lifespan, which means the supply of EPA to the brain must be constantly renewed. As a result, when you do a post-mortem analysis of the brain to look for EPA, it simply isn't there compared to the longer-lived AA and DHA present in the phospholipids of the brain. It is the ultimate disappearing act in nature.

Eicosanoids: Good and Bad

Five hundred million years ago, the only life forms on the planet were single-celled organisms. The explosion of biological diversity that created multi-cellular organisms required a new form of communication to allow cells with different functions to communicate within this more complex organism. That communication system was based on hormones, which acted as messengers in the early beginnings of the biological Internet. Eicosanoids were the first hormones developed by living organisms; they had to do a lot of multi-tasking in the early days of the first multi-celled organisms. That's why eicosanoids remain at the apex of the hormonal control mechanisms that directly or indirectly control all other hormonal actions in the body.

As with any good control system, you need an effective system of checks and balances. That's why there are "good" eicosanoids and "bad" eicosanoids. These hormones are not good or bad in the absolute sense but simply have powerful yet opposing biological actions. Relative to inflammation, bad eicosanoids initiate (or turn on) inflammatory responses, and good eicosanoids resolve (that is, turn off) inflammatory responses. As long as these are balanced, the body's inflammatory responses can respond to microbial attack or physical injuries quickly and will also bring the inflammatory response back to homeostasis as rapidly as possible.

The enzymes that convert omega-6 and omega-3 fatty acids into eicosanoids are diverse. Two of these—COX and LOX enzymes—have already been mentioned. But this is only a small number of the enzymes available to generate a wide number of different eicosanoids. The key factor is that both omega-6 and omega-3 fatty acids compete for these same enzymes. It is like a biological lottery: If you have the correct balance of these essential fatty acids in the cell, you win as the cell's inflammatory response is in balance. If you have an excess of omega-6 to omega-3 fatty acids in the cell, then you run the risk of chronic low-level inflammation that leads to obesity, chronic disease, and the acceleration of the aging process.

The Innate Immune System

You might think that the most primitive part of our immune system would be the simplest to figure out. After all, it is very similar to the immune system in plants. It turns out such thinking is wrong. Although the innate immune system is ancient, it is also very complex. That's why the 2011 Nobel Prize in Medicine was awarded for earlier discoveries that began to unlock its sophisticated control mechanisms for maintaining an appropriate inflammatory response.

The innate immune system is relatively non-specific because it recognizes fragments of invading microbes that are taken as signals that the cell may be under attack. Once a microbial fragment is recognized, a complex series of signaling reactions take place that result in the release of a wide variety of inflammatory proteins. These inflammatory proteins can either be new inflammatory signaling proteins (cytokines such as TNF, IL-1, and IL-6) that interact with nearby cells to stimulate their inflammatory responses or increased synthesis of inflammatory enzymes (COX-2) that can convert AA into pro-inflammatory eicosanoids that can transmit and amplify the inflammatory response to nearby cells.

Usually the first step in the process is the recognition of the fragments by sensors on the surface of the cell, known as toll-like receptors. (They were first discovered in fruit flies, as their absence made the fruit flies look weird. The German word for weird is *toll*). If you have a leaky gut, then you have a high likelihood of bacteria or bacteria fragments leaking into the blood. The toll-like receptors recognize these fragments as an indication you are under microbial attack and initiate the release of powerful inflammatory responses via the innate immune system. Unfortunately, these biological sentinels aren't very discriminating, and as a result, food molecules can also interact with them. As an example, toll-like receptor 4 (TLR-4) recognizes a saturated fatty acid component of the bacterial wall. Dietary saturated fats can also bind to this same TLR-4 sensor and induce an inflammatory response.

The next step in the process is the interaction of the signals coming from activated toll-like receptors with specialized proteins inside the cell known as gene transcription factors, also found in every cell. These are the key players that turn on and turn off gene expression. The two most important from the standpoint of cellular inflammation are nuclear factor kappaB (NF-κB) and peroxisomal proliferator activator gamma (PPAR-γ). NF-κB is the genetic master switch that turns on inflammation, while PPAR-γ turns off the generation of inflammation by inhibiting NF-κB. Anything (including food components, such as saturated fats) that activates toll-like receptors will activate NF-κB. Likewise, anything (including food components such as omega-3 fatty acids and polyphenols) that activates PPAR-γ will reduce inflammation. However, the most powerful activator of NF-κB is stimulated by a group of inflammatory eicosanoids (leukotrienes and hydroxylated fatty acids such as 12-HETE) derived from AA. The more you lower AA in your cell membranes as well as increase the levels of EPA and DHA, the less likely you are to activate NF-κB. You reduce the levels of AA and saturated fat by following the Mediterranean

Zone. You increase EPA and DHA by eating a lot of fatty fish or taking purified omega-3 fatty acid supplements.

Another activator of NF-κB is oxidative stress, usually the consequence of excess free radical production. Excess glucose in the blood is a significant driver of oxidative stress because it is so chemically reactive. This is why excess carbohydrates as well as excess omega-6 and saturated fats are dietary factors that increase cellular inflammation.

Although activation of PPAR-γ can inhibit the activation of NF-κB that starts the inflammation process, it can't inhibit the inflammatory mediators (cytokines) that are released once NF-κB has caused the expression of inflammatory genes. Returning these inflammatory dogs of war to their barracks is done during the resolution phase of inflammation.

Inflammation doesn't stop like the embers of a burning log dying out. It will continue unless reversed by an equally complex resolution response. This is driven primarily by a group of pro-resolution eicosanoids derived from omega-3 fatty acids called resolvins. Without adequate levels of omega-3 fatty acids in the diet, it is difficult to make adequate levels of resolvins. As a consequence, the soldiers of your immune response now start attacking normal tissue. This leads to long-term organ damage that, if severe enough, we call it chronic disease. My molecular definition of wellness is the maintenance of the balance of the initiation and resolution phases of inflammation in a tightly regulated zone.

One of the consequences of the increased release of inflammatory mediators is the activation of the killer cells (neutrophils and macrophages) of the innate immune system. These killer cells are the normally benign white cells of the circulatory system. However, they are quickly transformed into rogue killing machines once inflammatory mediators such as cytokines or eicosanoids activate them. One of the primary ways that these rogue warrior cells can attack microbial invaders is by the generation of free radicals, which act as localizing radiation. To minimize damage to normal tissue, another key safety valve to control the oxidative damage caused by these excess free radicals is to signal for more anti-oxidant enzymes to be produced. This is done by the interaction of polyphenols with the gene transcription factor Nrf2 that causes the increased synthesis of additional anti-oxidant proteins such as superoxide dismutase (SOD) and glutathione peroxides (GPX) to neutralize any continuing flow of excess free radicals from the immune cells, which may not realize their mission is over and they are no longer needed.

If you want to control cellular inflammation, you have to decrease certain types of fats (omega-6 and saturated fats) in the diet as well as the hormones (such as insulin) stimulated by high-glycemic carbohydrates that can stimulate a hair-trigger inflammatory response by accelerating AA formation. You lower AA formation by eating a lot of non-starchy vegetables with limited amounts of fruits and using only fats low in omega-6 fatty acids (such as olive oil). At the same time, you have to increase the levels of omega-3 fats and polyphenols to be able to resolve the inflammation. If this sounds like the Mediterranean Zone, it is.

Cellular Inflammation: A Chronic Imbalance of Inflammation and Resolution

The molecular definition of cellular inflammation is an imbalance in pro-inflammatory responses and the resolution of inflammation leading to chronic low-level activation of inflammation.

There are two types of inflammation. The first type is classical inflammation, which generates easily observed inflammatory responses, such as heat, redness, swelling, pain, and eventually loss of organ function. The other type is cellular inflammation, which is below the perception of pain and is more deadly because it can linger unnoticed and unaddressed for years, if not decades, constantly damaging organ function. Cellular inflammation can be caused by either (1) *excess* AA formation that turns *on* the innate immune system, or (2) a *deficiency* of EPA and DHA that turns *off* an activated innate immune system. In either case, if these on-off commands are imbalanced, your body is at long-term risk of developing a chronic disease at an earlier age. Furthermore, increased cellular inflammation disrupts hormonal signaling networks throughout the body. This is the cause of hormonal resistance, and in particular insulin resistance. As a result, you gain weight, develop chronic disease more rapidly, and age faster.

Dietary Modulation of Cellular Inflammation

Anti-inflammatory nutrition is based on the ability of certain nutrients to reduce the activation of NF-κB. The most effective way to lower the activation of NF-κB is to reduce the levels of AA in the target cell membrane, reducing the formation of leukotrienes and hydroxylated fatty acids, which can activate NF-κB. Following the Mediterranean Zone to reduce insulin levels coupled with the simultaneous lowering of the intake of omega-6 fatty acids is the primary lifelong dietary strategy to achieve and maintain a healthy, balanced inflammatory response.

Another effective dietary approach (and often easier to comply with) to reduce cellular inflammation is the enhancement of the resolution process of inflammation. This can be accomplished by dietary supplementation with adequate levels of purified high-dose fish oil rich in omega-3 fatty acids, such as EPA and DHA. Taken at high enough levels, these omega-3 fatty acids will lower AA levels somewhat (EPA more than DHA because it is more structurally similar to AA), but also dramatically increase EPA levels, which leads to increased resolvin production. The impact of this dietary change is reflected in the AA/EPA ratio in the blood (and therefore in the cell membranes of your various organs). This will have several anti-inflammatory benefits. First, a low AA/EPA ratio in the blood will reduce the likelihood of the formation of inflammatory eicosanoids derived from AA that can activate NF-κB. This is because leukotrienes derived from AA are pro-inflammatory, whereas those leukotrienes from EPA are non-inflammatory. Second, the increased intake of both EPA and DHA can activate the anti-inflammatory gene transcription factor PPAR-γ inside the cell as well as decrease the binding of saturated fatty acids to TLR-4 on the cell surface. Third, and most important, is the increased levels of resolvins derived from EPA and DHA will dramatically accelerate the resolution process of inflammation. This illustrates the multi-functional roles that omega-3 fatty acids have in controlling cellular inflammation.

The third dietary intervention to reduce diet-induced inflammation is the adequate intake of dietary polyphenols. Polyphenols are powerful anti-oxidants that at high enough levels reduce the formation of reactive oxygen species (ROS) that are generated by the conversion of dietary calories into chemical energy as well as the ROS generated by activated immune cells, such as neutrophils and macrophages. Excess ROS can activate NF-κB. Polyphenols can also inhibit the activation of NF-κB by activating the anti-inflammatory gene transcription factor (PPAR-γ), making poly-phenols both anti-oxidants and anti-inflammatory compounds.

Finally, the least effective dietary strategy—but still a useful one—is reducing the intake of saturated fat. (The American Heart Association was partially right about reducing the intake of saturated fat, but for the wrong reason.) This is because saturated fatty acids will cause the activation of the TLR-4 receptor in the cell membrane. (Remember this toll-like receptor binds to saturated fats and activates NF-κB.)

Obviously, the greater the number of these dietary strategies that you employ in your daily life, the greater their overall effect in reducing diet-induced inflammation. The easiest way to make them all come together at the same time is by following the Mediterranean Zone on a lifetime basis.

Since cellular inflammation (chronic activation of NF-κB) is confined to the cell itself, there are no blood markers that can be used to directly measure it. However, there are indirect ways to measure cellular inflammation. The commonly used marker of high-sensitivity C-reactive protein (hs-CRP) is not a very good indicator because it is highly sensitive to slight increases in bacterial infection and only increases after long-term activation of NF-κB. On the other hand, the AA/EPA ratio in the blood indicates that a tipping point has been reached that is likely to activate NF-κB in the cells. Consider the AA/EPA ratio to be your early-warning system for increased cellular inflammation—an elevated level of the AA/EPA ratio often precedes the development of elevated hs-CRP by several years, if not decades.

Chronic Disease

Ultimately you want to control levels of cellular inflammation to retard the development of chronic disease and, in the process, slow down the aging process.

Under ideal conditions, the initiation phase of inflammation is counterbalanced by the resolution phases of inflammation. This can be measured by the AA/EPA ratio in the blood. If the AA/EPA ratio is high, this indicates that your ability to resolve inflammation is compromised. The body has a fail-safe mechanism to solve this problem. It's called fibrosis. Think of fibrosis as burying toxic waste. If your body can't adequately resolve the inflammatory process, then it can just bury it by cementing it over with scar tissue. You contain the inflammation, but you damage that area of the organ. Scar tissue on the surface of the skin is a visual indication of what is taking place during fibrosis inside your body. Observing internal scarring is more difficult, but the loss of organ function that comes with extensive fibrosis is not. Atherosclerotic plaques are the result of fibrosis, for instance. If those plaques are not completely encased by a fibrous cap enriched in calcium, they can rupture, leading to sudden cardiac death. Or if you have too much scar tissue in the heart, it fails to function, and we call it heart failure. Cirrhosis of the liver is the result of extensive fibrosis. If the liver doesn't function because of extensive fibrosis, it is called liver failure, requiring a lifetime of dialysis or a liver transplant. Chronic obstructive pulmonary disease (COPD) is a result of fibrous lung tissue. The list goes on. The reason for fibrosis is the failure of the resolution response to work properly in the first place. The more fibrosis you have in the body, the less effectively your organs work and that is what we call aging.

It is now becoming recognized that virtually every chronic disease condition starts with either an increased initiation or a reduced resolution of the inflammatory response. In fact, it might be more correct to state that chronic disease is not *caused* by inflammation, but is really a *consequence* of the lack of adequate resolution. The more these two separate parts of the inflammatory response are imbalanced, the greater the production of cellular inflammation. The better able we are to control cellular inflammation, and the longer we put off the development of chronic disease, the longer and better you are going to live. The Mediterranean Zone provides a clear path to that goal.

Appendix C

Inflammation and Obesity

The definition of *obesity* is "the accumulation of excess body fat," not excess weight. In practical terms, we usually identify obesity by how we look stark naked in the mirror. However, it is the excess fat accumulation in our organs that we can't see that ultimately determines how detrimental that obesity will be to our future health. This is called lipotoxicity and is the first step toward developing diabetes. But first let's start with two very separate questions: (1) How do we get fat? (2) Why do we get fat?

HOW WE GET FAT

Although the diet book industry is devoted to weight loss, no one seems to be quite able to describe how we actually get fat. I described the process in greater detail in my book *Toxic Fat*, but here is a short summary.

Your fat cells are the only cells in the body that can safely store fat; and if they are healthy fat cells, that is exactly what they will do. By removing excess fatty acids from the bloodstream, your fat cells prevent lipotoxicity. This is the scientific term for when fat goes to all the wrong places, such as your liver, your muscles, or your heart cells, for example. As I stated earlier in this book, insulin is the central hormonal hub of your metabolism. Because high levels of lipids in the blood are toxic, insulin plays a key role in removing them and storing them safely in your fat calls. How insulin aids in helping your fat cells to remove excess blood fat is a little more complicated than simply saying "insulin makes you fat."

Your fat cells are sensitive to insulin, as it is needed to increase the transport of glucose from the blood into your fat cells. Once in the fat cells, the glucose is converted to glycerol, which by itself will not remove any excess fat from the blood. However, insulin also can increase the release of free fatty acids from lipoproteins passing by the fat cells by the stimulating enzyme (lipoprotein lipase) that sits at the surface of the blood vessels that surround the fat cells. This increases the amount of free fatty acids, but these require fatty acid binding proteins to transport the newly released fatty acids into the fat cells. The production of those fatty acid binding proteins is also stimulated by insulin. Once you have both glycerol and fatty acids together within the fat cell, they can recombine to form triglycerides for long-term safe storage. The more fat and carbohydrates (especially high-glycemic carbohydrates that stimulate insulin secretion) you consume, the more fat you will store in the fat cells. This is how high insulin levels make you fat. In this case, insulin acts as a safety hormone to prevent a lipid overload in the bloodstream.

When you are not eating (such as during sleep), the fat storage process in healthy fat cells begins to reverse itself. As insulin levels drop, an enzyme in the fat cells splits the stored triglycerides back into fatty acids and glycerol to be released into the bloodstream. The fatty acids go to other cells throughout the body to be converted into chemical energy (that is, ATP) in their mitochrondria (these are the parts of the cell that convert dietary calories into ATP) to get you through the starvation period, and the glycerol is converted into glucose for the brain. Under normal conditions, when fat cells are healthy, your adipose tissue acts as a bank. You make deposits during the day and withdrawals at night. Of course, if you are maintaining high levels of insulin all the time, then you are inhibiting the key step required to release stored fat to be used as energy. This is why high levels of insulin keep you fat.

There is a small percentage of obese individuals (5 to 8 percent) who are actually quite healthy regardless of their level of obesity. They are termed "metabolically healthy obese." My definition of metabolically healthy obese is based on the Edmonton Obesity Scoring System (EOSS). This is a much more rigid definition of *healthy* than usually used by researchers. More important, those obese individuals who are truly healthy by the EOSS definition remain healthy for many years. On the other hand, if you are obese and have even one indicator of adverse health (high blood pressure, elevated lipid levels, or elevated blood glucose), then you will see a statistically significant decrease in your eventual health over an extended period of time. The truly "metabolically healthy" have lots of healthy fat cells. While they may not look good in a swimsuit, they are able to store excess fat safely and not have it spread like cancer to other organs in their bodies.

So how do you explain the common theme in diet books that eating carbohydrates makes you fat? After all, the amount of glucose entering the fat cells facilitated by insulin is very limited. Is it possible that eating a lot of carbohydrates can be converted into circulating fat? The answer is yes, through a process known as lipogenesis, which takes place in the liver. As you might expect, certain gene transcription factors play an important role in this process. In particular, it is the carbohydrate response element binding protein (ChREBP), which is activated by glucose, that is the key player. The higher the carbohydrate content of your diet, the more glucose will enter into your liver. Higher levels of glucose activate ChREBP, which when coupled with increased insulin stimulates the synthesis of key enzymes needed to convert carbohydrates to fatty acids. The increased amounts of fatty acids are then reassembled in the liver into lipoproteins that can enter the bloodstream. If levels of these newly synthesized lipoproteins rise too rapidly, insulin will go into action to transfer those fatty acids for safe storage in the fat cells as described above. This is why the current Mediterranean diet has little effect on weight loss. It is simply too high in carbohydrates (especially high-glycemic carbohydrates) to reduce the secretion of insulin and activation of ChREBP.

The obvious solution is to reduce insulin levels, keeping in mind you need some insulin, but not too much, to run a smoothly functioning metabolism. The worst way to manage insulin levels is to simply eat protein with very little fat or carbohydrate. The first step of protein metabolism is its conversion to urea. But without adequate levels of fats or carbohydrates to aid the continued metabolism of urea to less toxic products, it builds up in the blood, leading to a condition known as rabbit starvation. (Early Arctic explorers who ate only very lean meat, such as rabbits, suffered from this condition.) Anytime the protein levels of the diet exceed more than 40 percent of total calories, the possibility the rapid buildup of urea in the blood will exist. Slightly less dangerous, but definitely not optimal, is the replacement of much of the carbohydrate in the diet with fat as in ketogenic diets such as the Atkins diet. Yes, you will reduce insulin levels, but now what are you going to do with all that extra fat in the blood? If you don't have enough insulin to drive that fat into fat cells, then the excess fat will go all the wrong places (lipotoxicity), usually starting with the liver. The more desirable approach is to reduce the levels of both fat *and* carbohydrate by restricting calories, yet keeping the amounts of carbohydrates and fat relatively balanced so the liver maintains flexibility in the production of the different sets of enzymes necessary for the efficient metabolic processing of both nutrients. Furthermore, by reducing the absolute levels of both circulating carbohydrates and fat, you keep your fat metabolism running with the efficiency of a Swiss bank. To be even more effective, you want to add EPA and DHA to your diet as they not only inhibit ChREBP activity (decreasing lipogenesis) but also activate another gene transcription factor (PPAR-α) that drives fatty acids away from storage and toward oxidation. This is one time you can say, "It takes fat to burn fat," as long as that fat is rich in EPA and DHA. Of course, calorie restriction is only possible to maintain on a lifetime basis if you are never hungry, but more on that later in this appendix.

Unfortunately, this elegant system starts to run amok when there is increased cellular inflammation in the fat cells. If you are eating a high-glycemic load diet coupled with high levels of omega-6 fatty acids, AA levels will start building up in the blood. AA along with the other fatty acids in the blood will be taken up by the fat cells through the action of insulin. But as the levels of AA begin to increase in the fat cells, so does cellular inflammation. Now otherwise healthy fat cells start becoming sick fat cells. One of the first consequences of the increase in cellular inflammation is the partial inhibition of a key enzyme (insulin-sensitive lipase) that releases stored fat as insulin levels drop. The release of stored fat, instead of being inhibited by insulin, is being continually released back into the bloodstream because the insulin signaling is being disrupted by the growing cellular inflammation in the fat cell. If your uptake mechanism for removing newly released fatty acids from the fat cells into the blood is saturated (as it will be by eating a high-fat diet), then these constantly released fatty acids from the fat cells begin to get deposited in other organs such as the liver and the muscles cells. As the levels of fat increase inside these organs, their ability to respond to insulin's signal to take up glucose from the blood also becomes compromised. Now you get insulin resistance in these cells (especially if the fat being released from the fat cells is rich in AA), and glucose levels start to increase in the blood. Since excess blood glucose is also toxic to the body, the pancreas starts pumping more insulin into the bloodstream to try to bring down blood sugar levels. As insulin levels rise in the blood due to insulin resistance, a vicious cycle begins that causes accelerated storage of fat in the fat cells coupled with a growing lipotoxicity in other organs throughout the body. Obviously, this explanation is a little more complicated than making simple blanket statements that carbohydrates make you fat.

WHY DO WE GET FAT?

The obvious answer is that we eat more calories than we burn. Yes, calories do count. Any excess calories have to go somewhere. Excess carbs can be initially stored in the liver and the muscles, but those storage sites have a limited capacity. However, the excess carbohydrates can be converted to fat via lipogenesis, which takes place in the liver. Excess protein can only be stored in the muscle, but that is an even more limited process that requires consistent weight training to release growth hormone from the pituitary gland. Consumption of excess protein without the presence of growth hormone will simply be metabolized into glucose (via neoglucogenesis) or fat. On the other hand, excess dietary fat can be indefinitely stored in our fat cells since these cells have the ability to expand dramatically. So if you eat more calories than the body needs to maintain its metabolism, it is quite likely that, with the help of insulin, these extra calories will end up in your fat cells.

But the question is *why* are people eating more calories today? I believe the answer is simple: We are hungrier because the biological Internet that tells the brain we have more than sufficient calories to maintain our metabolism has been disrupted. As you might expect, the suspect is increased cellular inflammation.

According to the USDA, Americans were eating 474 more calories per day in 2010 than in 1970. That alone is sufficient to explain the increase in obesity. What is more ominous is that more than 90 percent of those increased calories come from added fats and oils (48 percent), grains (38 percent), and sugar and sweeteners (7 percent). Those numbers suggest that if you are looking for a likely suspect for increased obesity, grains and fats are the most likely suspects, not the much smaller increase in the consumption of sugar and sweeteners over the past forty years. Grains (including whole grains) are high-glycemic load carbohydrates that are 100 percent composed of glucose. As they rapidly enter the bloodstream (often faster than sugar), increased insulin secretion is a guaranteed consequence. Many of the added fats are rich in omega-6 fatty acids. With these two food ingredients, you have a surefire metabolic prescription to increase cellular inflammation through the increased production of AA. So why would increased cellular inflammation make you hungry? To understand that, it is necessary to explore the complex science of how our hormones actually control hunger.

Let's start with insulin. If you consume too many high-glycemic load carbohydrates, then blood glucose levels rapidly rise. Because blood glucose is toxic at high levels, the body responds by secreting insulin to drive excess blood glucose into your fat, muscle, and liver cells.

If the rise in blood glucose is too rapid, then there is often an oversecretion of insulin, and then blood glucose levels drop too low, leading to hypoglycemia. This is what happens when you eat a big meal of pasta at noon, and two hours later you have a difficult time keeping your eyes open. To address the low blood glucose problem caused by consuming high-glycemic load carbohydrates, the brain implores you to begin searching for any high-glycemic food (candy bar, chips, or ideally a sugar-laden soda) that can quickly restore the low blood glucose levels. The use of these foods becomes a way of self-medicating to elevate low blood glucose levels. This may explain why the most popular spot in a hospital at the end of a work shift is the vending machine.

However, if you can't find a convenient source of glucose to quickly restore blood sugar levels, then the brain has an alternative mechanism to do so: increasing cortisol secretion to break down muscle into glucose via a process known as neo-glucogenesis. This is what happens when you follow ketogenic low-carbohydrate diets such as the Atkins diet. The common party line for advocates of ketogenic diets is that the brain prefers ketones to glucose for energy. I simply don't buy that argument. Even under total starvation conditions, the brain levels of glucose never drop to less than 40 mg/dl due to neo-glucogenesis. At lower blood glucose levels (such as 25 to 35 mg/dl), the brain goes into lethargy, convulsions, and potentially a coma. If ketones generated by ketogeneic diets were such great sources of energy for the brain, then theoretically blood glucose levels could drop to zero and the brain would be completely happy.

Researchers at Harvard Medical School demonstrated that cortisol levels increased by 18 percent after three months on the Atkins diet. Some of the consequences of increased cortisol levels are (1) you are hungrier (due to increased insulin resistance), (2) sicker (due to depressed immune function), and (3) less mentally sharp (due to destruction of neurons in the hippocampus region of the brain by their continuing exposure to excess cortisol). Three pretty good reasons to maintain adequate levels of blood glucose—not too much so the body secretes more insulin to reduce potentially toxic glucose levels in the blood, but not too little, which would cause the overproduction of cortisol in order to produce enough glucose for the brain.

However, insulin and cortisol are only two of many hormones that are key in the control of hunger and satiety. Some of the other hormones in this complex orchestration of appetite are listed below.

Hunger Hormones	Satiety Hormones
Cortisol	Leptin
Endocannabinoids	CCK
Ghrelin	PYY
Insulin (in the blood)	Insulin (in the brain)
NPY	GLP-1

The activation of satiety and hunger neurons is affected by a number of different hormones sending in information from diverse locations throughout the body. This complexity is best illustrated by how insulin works. High levels of insulin in the blood lower blood glucose levels. This makes you hungry because the brain is now deprived of its primary source of energy. If the brain is hungry, then you will be hungry. However, inside the brain it is a different story. Once insulin enters the brain, it can inhibit the stimulation of the hunger neurons, thus increasing satiety. (This is why if you push insulin levels too low by eating too few calories or not enough carbohydrates, you get hungry again.) What prevents insulin from signaling the brain to stop looking for food is insulin resistance. The same is true for the hormone leptin, which is produced in your fat cells. The more excess body fat you have, the more leptin you generate. Theoretically, if leptin can get to the brain, obese individuals will stop eating. Unfortunately, the same cellular inflammation that generates insulin resistance in the brain also generates leptin resistance. To overcome both insulin resistance and leptin resistance in the central nervous system, you have to reduce cellular inflammation if you want to increase satiety. This is why hunger is really a consequence of increased cellular inflammation, not decreased willpower. Fortunately, both insulin and leptin resistance can be reduced by following the Mediterranean Zone, which balances both hunger and satiety hormones so that you are not hungry for five hours after a meal.

Ultimately, much of the hormonal action that regulates hunger takes place in the brain, specifically at the base of the hypothalamus. Within this part of the hypothalamus are both appetite-stimulating (hunger) and appetite-suppressing (satiety) neurons. Hormones such as neuropeptide Y (NPY) stimulate the hunger neurons, whereas peptide YY (PYY) stimulate the satiety neurons. Depending upon which set of neurons is activated, an integrated signal is sent to another part of the hypothalamus that ultimately determines whether you should eat or not. Sound complicated? Yes, but that is only part of the issue.

Although the digestive system is a great distance from the brain, it also plays a significant role in the control of both hunger and satiety. The hormone ghrelin is activated by the lack of food in the stomach. Its release from the stomach goes directly to the brain to activate the hunger neurons. However, PYY (stimulated by dietary protein) is secreted from the ileum (the lower part of the small intestine) and the upper part of the colon (the large intestine) to inhibit the action of ghrelin secreted by the stomach. This provides a nice on-off system to signal to the brain from different parts of the digestive system as to when to start and stop eating. Obese individuals have reduced levels of PYY, which means they have a reduced "off" switch when it comes to appetite control. Other gut-based hormones such as GLP-1 and CCK also aid in the satiety mechanism.

Control of hunger is a consequence of the dynamic balance of these and other hormones in the blood, gut, and brain. Making it even more difficult to lose weight and keep it off is the fact that the body goes to great efforts to defend the loss of excess body fat. For example, when you lose weight by dieting, the levels of the hunger hormone ghrelin increase and the levels of the satiety hormone PYY decrease. This makes trying to cut back on calories by simply using willpower to try to eat less such a difficult process.

The last major hormonal players in the brain that can override this intricate balance of external endocrine hormones on the satiety and hunger neurons are the endocannabinoids. Anyone who has had the experience of smoking marijuana knows one of its most immediate side effects is increased hunger ("the munchies"); the active ingredient in marijuana (tetrahydrocannabinol, or THC) interacts with these endocannabinoid receptors in the brain that make you incredibly hungry. These hunger-inducing hormones interact in a different part of the hypothalamus to regulate appetite. Since the natural endocannabinoids in your brain are derived from AA, the more AA you produce by your diet, the hungrier you become. One of the most important benefits of the Mediterranean Zone is that you are not as hungry. Why? You are reducing the production of endocannabinoids by reducing the formation of AA. This is why the Mediterranean Zone places a strong emphasis in keeping omega-6 fatty acids as low as possible as well as reducing the glycemic load of the diet. Those two factors will reduce excess levels of AA in the body and the brain.

Another way to reduce elevated endocannabinoid levels is to also make sure that you are consuming adequate levels of omega-3 fatty acids (either by eating a lot of fish or taking purified omega-3 fatty acid supplements) to reduce the formation of endocannabinoids.

One final factor that can disrupt satiety signals is simply consuming too many calories at any one meal, which causes metabolic inflammation in the hypothalamus. This is why I prefer the maximum calories at a meal to be 400 or less. All of the Mediterranean Zone meals presented earlier in this book contain less than 400 calories, yet supply adequate protein, carbohydrate, fat, vitamins, and minerals, and, most importantly, satiety.

Besides disrupting the hormonal communication that turns off satiety signals, increased production of AA also induces the development of new fat cells. This is known as adipogenesis. It has clearly been shown in animal models in which diets rich in omega-6 fatty acids and poor in omega-3 fatty acids are maintained for several generations. Each generation of the offspring becomes fatter than the previous even though the calorie intake remains constant. Epigenetic fetal programming may be the mechanism by which these events are generated. The same trend appears to be happening to Americans.

There's no question that keeping weight from coming back after it has been lost is very difficult. Hormones in the gut are now working against you after weight loss. The appearance of appetizing food also excites the reward centers in the brain to a greater extent as a consequence of weight loss. You become hungrier and more preoccupied with food after losing weight. And your body becomes more efficient in converting dietary calories into energy, meaning you have to eat even less food to avoid regaining weight. Invariably, much of the lost weight is regained because of these biological mechanisms that defend against weight loss. Maybe this explains why the data on long-term weight control is so sparse, because people hate to admit to defeat. One source of data is the National Weight Control Registry, which is a self-selected group of individuals who have been successful in losing at least thirty pounds and keeping it off for more than a year. It appears that the use of a combination of long-term calorie restriction (less than 1,400 calories per day) coupled with an hour of exercise per day is probably needed for weight loss maintenance success. Since the National Weight Control Registry consists of only about ten thousand individuals since 1994, this might suggest that most people who lose weight have significant difficulty in keeping it off.

Currently the best way for losing weight and keeping it off is gastric bypass surgery. The most radical type of bypass surgery is known as Roux-en-Y, in which much of the small intestine is bypassed. As a result, the dietary components of your meal directly enter the ileum (the lower part of the small intestine), where the greatest concentrations of L-cells are located. The L-cells of the gut lining contain receptors for glucose and protein. If these receptors are activated, then hormonal signals to stop eating are sent directly to the brain via the vagal nerve. This is why if the carbohydrates (especially high-glycemic ones) and protein you are eating are quickly absorbed in the upper part of the intestine, there are less of these nutrients available to the L-cells in the lower part of the intestine. Therefore, the body is less likely to release the necessary hormonal "stop-eating" signals to the brain. As a result, you are constantly hungry. On the other hand, with the gastric re-routing by bypass surgery, more of the ingested food is being delivered to the lower part of the intestine. In particular, the levels of PYY and GLP-1 are increased and levels of ghrelin are decreased. Gastric-bypass patients get immediate freedom from hunger on the first day. That's why they can maintain long-term weight loss.

The Mediterranean Zone provides an effective and risk-free option for the holy grail of long-term weight control. You are consuming about 1,200 to 1,500 calories per day but without hunger. This is within the range of calorie consumption needed for long-term weight maintenance as indicated by the National Weight Control Registry. It does this by providing a significant increase in satiety using a variety of hormonal signaling strategies (using the balance of its food ingredients) to reduce cellular inflammation, as opposed to resorting to surgery and a lifetime of malnutrition.

Appendix D

Inflammation and

Chronic Disease

Under ideal conditions, the inflammatory response should be self-limiting, turning on only when it is needed and then turning itself off to return the body to homeostasis. This means the initiation phase of inflammation is balanced by the resolution phase of inflammation. Unfortunately, the real world never works so smoothly. When the balance of these two distinct phases of the inflammation is disrupted, the result is often a constant low-level cellular inflammation that accelerates the development of chronic disease conditions.

If the resolution process is not satisfactorily completed, the body builds scar tissue around the injured site to prevent any further access by the neutrophils and macrophages. This is called fibrosis, which will stop the continuing oxidative stress, but damages that localized area of the organ. When this happens consistently because your internal resolution response is too weak, you will eventually develop loss of organ function. This is the last expression of the classical cardinal signs of inflammation (heat, swelling, pain, redness, and loss of function). The first four occur quickly; the last (loss of function) takes time to develop.

Elevated cellular inflammation can also disturb the integral hormonal signaling pathways that control our metabolism. The most well known example of hormone resistance is insulin resistance, the poster child for the disruption of your biological Internet by cellular inflammation.

INSULIN RESISTANCE

Insulin resistance simply means that the metabolic signal of insulin to do something is not being correctly transmitted to its target inside the cell. Since a primary role of insulin is to reduce potentially toxic levels of glucose and fats in the blood in the presence of insulin resistance, the pancreas responds by secreting more insulin to try to reduce the levels of glucose and lipids in the blood by brute force. This results in hyperinsulinemia. What caused insulin resistance was a black box to researchers until the 1990s, when it was discovered that inflammatory cytokines (especially tumor necrosis factor, or TNF) seemed to be at the center of this disturbance. TNF is one of the inflammatory cytokines that is expressed once NF-κB is activated so it is reasonable to believe that insulin resistance may be a consequence of excess cellular inflammation. Not surprisingly, when you follow an anti-inflammatory diet such as the Mediterranean Zone, insulin resistance is reduced, which means that lower levels of insulin can do its job more effectively, and the hyperinsulinemia in the blood is reduced. That's why it is not surprising that the dietary guidelines of the Joslin Diabetes Research Center at Harvard Medical School for treating obesity, metabolic syndrome (pre-diabetes characterized by hyperinsulinemia), and diabetes are essentially that of the Zone Diet. The Mediterranean Zone simply takes those dietary recommendations to a much higher level of inflammatory control.

We often think of insulin resistance as being associated only with impaired insulin action in the liver and the muscles, but it really starts with the adipose tissue. In particular, the hormone-sensitive lipase, found in the fat cells, may be the first victim of insulin resistance. This enzyme controls the release of stored fats back into the bloodstream to be used as an energy source when insulin levels are low (such as when you are sleeping). With the development of insulin resistance, the stop signal of this enzyme, which is mediated by higher levels of insulin in the blood, becomes partially inhibited and fatty acids are now continuously released. Some of the fatty acids will be reabsorbed by the fat cells to be resynthesized into tri-glycerides, but the rest will now travel to other organs such as the liver and muscle cells. If those fatty acids are rich in AA, then they become delivery agents for spreading cellular inflammation to these organs. As insulin re-sistance spreads to these organs, they, too, become resistant to insulin's action, requiring the pancreas to secrete ever-increasing levels of insulin to bring down potentially toxic levels of fats and glucose in the bloodstream. This explains why the levels of AA in the fat cells have a striking correla-tion with the increased likelihood of developing metabolic syndrome. The spread of stored AA because of insulin resistance in the fat cells simply speeds up the metastatic flow of cellular inflammation into other organs.

The extreme case of insulin resistance occurs in a condition known as lipodystrophy in which the fat cells are destroyed. Now the circulating fat in the blood has nowhere to be safely stored, and rapidly ends up in the liver and the muscles, causing significant insulin resistance. Lipodystrophy was a rare disease before the advent of AIDS. Unfortunately, the drugs that inhibit viral replication of the HIV virus also destroy fat cells. The result is a reprieve from an earlier death from AIDS, but a dramatic increase in insulin resistance eventually leading to diabetes and heart disease.

Insulin resistance doesn't always start out in the fat cells. There is some evidence from animal studies that ketogenic diets may force the circulat-ing fat into liver cells instead of being safely stored in fat cells because in-sulin levels are lowered too much.

Eventually, as insulin resistance increases, there is a corresponding in-crease in hyperinsulinemia that puts you in metabolic trouble. The hyper-insulinemia accelerates the deposition of circulating fat into your adipose tissue, decreasing the amount available to go to other tissues for conver-sion into energy. The result is that you become hungry and fatigued. In addition you accelerate the formation of AA by activating the key enzymes required to produce AA from omega-6 fatty acids, which increases cellular inflammation in every cell in your body.

As you develop insulin resistance in the liver and muscle, you are also beginning to develop insulin and leptin resistance in the hypothalamus. As a consequence, both insulin and leptin (which act as satiety signals) are not recognized and hunger increases. As you eat more calories to try to satisfy your hunger, you gain more body fat due to increasing hyperinsulinemia. In addition, the excess calories also cause increased inflammation in the hypothalamus, which further increases hunger by interfering with incoming satiety signals.

If left untreated, metabolic syndrome eventually becomes type 2 diabetes. This usually occurs within ten to twenty years after the initial diagnosis. The insulin producing beta cells of the pancreas simply become exhausted by the continued demand to make more insulin to control the ever-increasing levels of blood glucose. It appears part of this exhaustion is due to the infiltration of macrophages that attack the beta cells. As the pancreas becomes less able to produce insulin, the blood glucose levels begin to skyrocket, increasing the levels of oxidative stress throughout the body. Oxidative stress activates NF-κB, and cellular inflammation increases correspondingly. With the development of diabetes comes a host of other inflammation-related diseases, such as heart disease, Alzheimer's, ocular disorders, kidney failure, neuropathy, and impaired wound healing (which can lead to infection, gangrene, and eventually amputation). Not a very pleasant picture.

One of the first consequences of insulin resistance in the liver cells is the disruption of lipoprotein metabolism. Small dense LDL particles (which are highly prone to becoming oxidized LDL particles) begin to accumulate, HDL particles begin to decrease, and triglycerides (TG) levels begin to rise. This is why the TG/HDL cholesterol ratio is a sensitive indicator of developing insulin resistance in the liver that results in a fatty liver. The development of non-alcoholic steatohepatitis (NASH) is usually the first step in this fatty liver disease. Left untreated, this can eventually progress to cirrhosis (caused by increasing scar damage due to the unresolved inflammation) and eventually liver failure if organ function is totally compromised by fibrosis.

The small dense LDL particles produced by an inflamed liver are more prone to oxidation because of their size. They are also more likely to begin to accumulate in the heart cells, generating atherosclerotic lesions. Oxidized LDL particles can readily circumvent the normal uptake mechanism of non-oxidized LDL particles that is self-regulating as the cell senses it has adequate levels of cholesterol and shuts down any further uptake of normal LDL particles. On the other hand, the oxidized LDL particles are rapidly taken up by macrophages in the atherosclerotic lesion in the form of the classic lipid-laden foam cells, which are more prone to rupture. This helps explain why heart disease is highly correlated with metabolic syndrome and why elevated levels of AA in the adipose tissue are also correlated with increasing heart disease.

However, the real cause of mortality from heart disease is not lipid accumulation, but the rupture of the atherosclerotic plaque. The primary culprits are soft vulnerable plaques. They are called soft because they have not been encased in a thick fibrosis cap rich in calcium that makes it difficult for a hard plaque to rupture. These vulnerable soft plaques can't be detected with scanning techniques such as CAT scans that easily pick up calcium deposits in the hard plaques. As a result, the soft plaques are all but invisible to CAT scans. Since they have no fibrous cap, they can easily rupture if the levels of cellular inflammation within them become too elevated. The ruptured plaque releases cellular debris that causes rapid formation of a clot in the artery that causes the stoppage of blood flow and often results in sudden cardiac death.

Strokes can be viewed as "brain attacks" because cerebral arteries develop the lesions as opposed to the cardiovascular arteries. While the location of the soft vulnerable plaques may be different in a different area (the cerebral artery as opposed to the vascular system), the molecular mechanism behind their development is similar as in heart disease.

Cancer is often viewed as genetic disease; however, I believe it can be better understood as a metabolic and inflammatory disease. Rarely will the primary tumor cause death. However, if the primary tumor metastasizes to other organs, the eventual outcome for the patient is often bleak. What mediates that metastasis is inflammation, and in particular inflammatory eicosanoids derived from AA. These eicosanoids (especially PGE_2) depress the local inflammatory responses that would otherwise help orchestrate the destruction of the cancer cell, and other eicosanoids (hydroxylated fatty acids such as 12-HETE) derived from AA help the circulating tumor cells to get a foothold in a new location. In fact, cancer is often described as "a wound that never heals." That is also a good definition of unresolved inflammation. One of the inflammatory factors released by the activation of NF-κB is a group of enzymes known as matrix metalloproteinases (MMP) that break down the collagen matrix, making it easier for a roaming tumor cell in the blood to enter a new site. Both events are enhanced by increased levels of AA in the cancer cell. The excess AA is transformed into leukotrienes that increase the activity of NF-κB that causes the synthesis of more

MMP and the excess AA is also the substrate required to make hydroxylated fatty acids and PGE_2, that facilitates metastasis.

The other factor that drives tumor cells is increased blood glucose levels. Tumor cells have a very limited capacity to oxidize fats for energy. They rely primarily on glucose to fuel their energy needs, so reducing blood glucose levels is an excellent metabolic strategy for managing tumor growth. In addition, high levels of blood glucose will increase insulin levels (especially in the presence of insulin resistance). Insulin is a growth factor and has significant cross-reactivity with another hormone—insulin-like growth factor, or IGF—that is a strong hormonal driver of tumor cell growth. This is not to say that genetic factors are not important in cancer, but only to note that you have a great ability to control your metabolism by an anti-inflammatory diet to make it much more difficult for tumors to grow and metastasize.

Many of the chronic diseases that are the result of immunological disturbances can be broken down into two categories: conditions driven by fibrosis, and those driven by unresolved inflammation.

Chronic pulmonary obstructive disease (COPD) has quickly risen to be the third leading cause of death after heart disease and cancer in the United States. Obviously initiated by pulmonary inflammation, it ends with loss of lung function caused by extensive fibrosis as a result of lack of resolution of the inflammation response. With COPD, you eventually require supplemental oxygen to maintain minimal oxygen levels in the blood. Other chronic diseases that fall into this category include liver failure (which requires a transplant) and kidney failure (which requires constant dialysis). All three diseases can be considered examples of failure of the resolution process and forcing that particular organ into the fallback strategy of scar tissue formation. With time, repeated inflammatory attacks leads to further loss of organ function.

Other immunological diseases, such as arthritis, systematic pain (such as fibromyalgia), gut disorders (Crohn's disease and ulcerative colitis), allergies, asthma, and a wide number of other immunological disorders can also be considered as examples of unresolved resolution, but without the fibrosis. These diseases are usually treated with constant application of anti-inflammatory drugs to take the place of the more optimal approach of the resolution of inflammation in the first place.

Finally, there are the neurological diseases, which, like immunological conditions, can be broken down into two distinct groups. The first is continued neuroinflammation without resolution. Diseases in this category include multiple sclerosis, Parkinson's, and Alzheimer's. The second category includes those neurological conditions that are the result of disrupted neurotransmitter communication between cells. You might consider these to be examples of neurotransmitter resistance, and these conditions would include depression, ADHD, and anxiety. As usual, the likely suspect in triggering these conditions is increased cellular inflammation.

This very brief overview suggests that the lack of inflammatory resolution may really be the root cause of most chronic diseases. Without adequate resolution, inflammation continues unabated at low chronic levels or the body resorts to an inferior option of fibrosis to reduce or contain the inflammation at a localized level. The primary treatment for reducing low-level cellular inflammation is not a drug, but an anti-inflammatory diet such as the Mediterranean Zone. The more you use the Mediterranean Zone as your primary drug of choice, the less you will need to rely upon pharmaceuticals to control the symptoms of chronic cellular inflammation.

Appendix E

Inflammation and Aging

The body is constantly renewing itself. Old or damaged tissue is being broken down, and new tissue is being made to take its place. If the old tissue is being broken down at a faster rate than new tissue is replacing it, then that mismatch in tissue renewal can be viewed as aging.

We can see the physical signs of aging in various locations in the body—the skin, the hair, bone loss, loss of muscle mass, increase in fat accumulation, and the loss of vision. What links all of these is increased cellular inflammation. So let's look at each of these visible signs of aging, and see what is really happening under the surface.

Skin

One of the first signs of aging is the loss of taut, plump, youthful skin. For most people, the appearance of wrinkles is the most disturbing sign of aging. Essentially, wrinkles can be best understood as biological potholes on the surface of the skin. They are the result of two factors: (1) the loss of fat in the dermis of the skin that thins the skin and (2) the breakdown of the collagen matrix that gives the skin its structural support. The result of this collagen degradation is a disorganized collagen fiber structural network. When coupled with the lack of dermal fat, the skin wrinkles. (This is why one of the hottest areas in dermatology is the injection of fat cells harvested from liposuction of one's own adipose tissue.) The ultimate cause of collagen destruction is the increased production of enzymes known as matrix metalloproteinases (MMP). You shouldn't be surprised that generation of these collagen-degrading proteins is a result of NF-κB activation. Externally, UV radiation increases the free radical formation that causes the activation of NF-κB. Sunscreens are good for blocking UVA radiation, but not as useful in stopping UVB radiation. Internally, an anti-inflammatory diet can inhibit the activation of NF-κB by both types of UV radiation. This is why the anti-inflammatory Mediterranean Zone, which is rich in polyphenols, can significantly reduce ROS (reactive oxygen species) production by UVB radiation as well as activating the gene transcription factor Nrf2, producing the increased synthesis of powerful anti-oxidant enzymes. It is also known that high levels of omega-3 fatty acids can inhibit the synthesis of MMP. Thus the Mediterranean Zone enriched with high-dose omega-3 fatty acids may represent the best "anti-aging prescription" for younger looking skin.

No one is quite sure what causes the loss of dermal fat. I suspect it may be due to insulin resistance inhibiting the action of insulin to keep fat stored in the dermal fat cells, thus reducing insulin resistance systemically, and helping to maintain dermal fat levels. The one thing I know for certain is that as you lose dermal fat, your sensitivity to cold significantly increases as you are losing a powerful thermal barrier, which would help retain your core temperature. This is why as people age, they often spend more time looking at travel brochures for potential winter travel in Florida, the Caribbean, and Mexico.

Hair

Hair loss is one of the facts of aging. Much of hair loss is genetically controlled, but there is an indication that those genetic predispositions may be altered by eicosanoids. In particular, the prostaglandin PGD_2 derived from AA inhibits hair growth. Another synthetic eicosanoid used to treat glaucoma can stimulate eyelash growth and is in preliminary studies for stimulating hair growth. Again, it is a matter of eicosanoid balance.

The loss of hair color is another obvious sign of aging. The latest research indicates that the graying of hair is due to the increased generation of ROS within the hair follicle. The best way to reduce ROS is to make sure you have high levels of polyphenols in the diet. Since ROS activates NF-κB, an anti-inflammatory diet coupled with high dose omega-3 fatty acids should also support maintaining hair color for longer periods of time.

Therefore, the best eicosanoid modulating and anti-oxidant "drug" for the hair may be the Mediterranean Zone coupled with high-dose fish oil.

Bone

You can live with wrinkles and gray hair, but loss of bone mass is another story. There are two types of cells in the bone: the osteoblasts that build bone and the osteoclasts that degrade and resorb bone. We tend to think that bone loss is due to lack of calcium, but in reality it is primarily a consequence of increased cellular inflammation that activates the osteoclasts. In animal models it has been shown that increasing the levels of omega-3 fatty acids provides a significant improvement in bone density. In particular, the resolvin derived from EPA (RvE1) has been shown to be effective in preventing bone resorption.

Loss of Muscle Mass

One reason that muscle mass decreases with age is the lowered levels of testosterone and growth hormone, which are the anabolic factors needed for maintenance of muscle for both men and women. This leads to sacro-penia (loss of muscle mass) and eventually frailty. Another factor leading to loss of muscle mass is the increase in pro-inflammatory cytokines that are produced as the result of increased cellular inflammation. Obviously, there is a continued need for exercise as a stimulus for creating new muscle mass. Even with the lowered levels of testosterone and growth hormone that comes with aging, this loss of muscle mass may be lessened by the reduction of inflammatory cytokines.

If you want to preserve muscle mass as you age, then ensuring that you have adequate protein intake and simultaneously reducing cellular inflammation are two dietary factors you can control. The Mediterranean Zone does it automatically for you. However, you still need to exercise on a daily basis to maintain testosterone and growth hormone levels. The greater the intensity of the exercise in short bursts (interval training), the better the results.

Increase in Body Fat

It's one thing to lose fat in your skin, but it is much more disturbing to gain fat in your abdomen and hips. This usually begins in your thirties even if your exercise and diet doesn't change that much from what it was in your twenties. This occurs because the levels of testosterone and estrogen—in both men and women—are dropping. Both of these hormones are very effective in preventing the accumulation of stored body fat in both males and females. Furthermore, as estrogen levels drop, insulin levels begin to increase, driving fat into the adipose tissue as opposed to diverting it to the peripheral tissues to make more ATP. Couple these facts with increasing insulin resistance caused by increased diet-induced inflammation and fat accumulation becomes a fact of aging. The best way to rectify the situation is calorie restriction without hunger or malnutrition. This is why if you want to look twenty years younger, your first step may be to lose 20 pounds of excess fat. If you are not overweight, then add 5 pounds of new muscle mass. The Mediterranean Zone provides such a pathway to reach either goal.

Loss of Vision

Vision loss is another obvious sign of aging. The primary cause of blindness after the age of 50 is age-related macular degeneration (AMD). The underlying cause of AMD is inflammation in the retina. In recently published work, I demonstrated that high-dose purified omega-3 fatty acids can reverse dry AMD (90 percent of all AMD is dry AMD), which is rather remarkable since there is no prescription drug capable of doing so. Subsequent analysis of the data demonstrates a strong relationship between the AA/EPA ratio and the gain of vision. For those with an AA/EPA ratio at 1.5, their gain of vision is twice as great as those with an AA/EPA ratio of 2.5. Considering that the average American has an AA/EPA of approximately 20, this means significant supplementation of omega-3 fatty acids would be needed to reduce cellular inflammation in the eye—a small price to pay for regaining your eyesight.

Transcription Factors

Any discussion of aging must include gene transcription factors, especially those that are important in metabolism. The two primary ones involved in aging appear to be mTOR (mammalian target of rapamycin) and AMP kinase. mTOR is the gene transcription factor that turns on growth and is directly activated by the amino acid leucine. It is essential for maintaining muscle mass. Unfortunately, it also stimulates tumor growth. AMP kinase is an energy sensor of ATP levels in the cell and acts as the master genetic switch of metabolism. If ATP levels are low, this enzyme is activated to recycle AMP back into ATP. At the same time it improves the efficiency of the general metabolism by slowing the anabolic process of tissue rebuilding that requires a lot of energy so that more ATP can be generated with fewer calories to maintain the functioning of existing cells. At the molecular levels, it is the constant balancing act of these two gene transcription factors that determines our rate of tissue renewal and the speed of aging.

Activation of mTOR for new protein synthesis is a consequence of the interaction of leucine to stimulate mTOR, coupled with the need for adequate insulin to drive nutrients into cells to provide the raw materials for new protein synthesis. On the other hand, AMP kinase can be activated by calorie restriction and polyphenols. Both act on the SIRT1 gene that is important in slowing the aging process. All of these factors are under your control. The Mediterranean Zone provides a blueprint to continually balance these two opposing gene transcription factors and thus control the rate of aging.

Successful Aging
Of course the primary problem with aging is the development of chronic disease (described in Appendix D), which robs us of our quality of life. So whether it is the slowing down of the development of chronic disease or simply reducing the physical signs of aging, both goals lead back to the reduction of diet-induced inflammation.

Appendix F

The Clinical Markers

of Wellness

We have many clinical markers of illness but relatively few markers of wellness. Ultimately, true health reform comes when patients take increased responsibility for their health by maintaining a state of wellness. The number-one factor within a patient's control is their diet because of its ability to manage cellular inflammation. However, with the rise of the industrialization and globalization of food, this is becoming a more difficult prospect on a worldwide level. Nonetheless, as I have shown throughout this book, it is actually quite easy to take control of your health care future by being in the Zone.

Being in the Zone is determined by clinical evidence, not hope. Your blood chemistry will tell you with absolute clarity whether you are in the Zone, and if not, you will have a clear indication from your test results what you have to do from a dietary standpoint to get there.

Broadly speaking, there are three distinct metabolic measurements that determine if you are in the Zone: (1) your levels of cellular inflammation, (2) your long-term control of blood sugar levels, and (3) your levels of insulin resistance. This is not a multiple-choice test. *Only when all three markers are in the appropriate ranges can you be considered to be in the*

Zone. Unfortunately, when we use those criteria, it appears that less than 1 percent of Americans can be considered to be well.

Cellular Inflammation

Since the Zone is about maintaining a healthy inflammatory response, your levels of cellular inflammation are an exceptionally important clinical marker.

Unfortunately, the most commonly used diagnostic marker of inflammation is C-reactive protein (CRP), which is simply not very reliable. CRP is a marker of long-term activation of NF-κB. Very few of the inflammatory mediators expressed in the cell by NF-κB can reach the blood. Most inflammatory mediators released by NF-κB act locally on nearby cells and enter the bloodstream with difficulty. Only one, IL-6, seems to have much success. Nonetheless, even IL-6 must eventually reach a very high level in the blood to interact with the liver to produce CRP. Since CRP is a more long-lived marker in the blood, it is much easier to measure than the more immediate inflammatory products (IL-1, IL-6, TNF, and COX-2 enzymes) produced by NF-κB activation. However, being easier to measure doesn't necessarily translate into a better clinical marker of cellular inflammation. In fact, an increased AA/EPA ratio in the blood often precedes any increase of C-reactive protein by several years, if not decades. An elevated AA/EPA ratio indicates that NF-κB is at the tipping point of chronic activation, and the cells in every organ in the body are primed for increased genetic expression of a wide variety of inflammatory mediators. The measurement of CRP only indicates that NF-κB has been activated for a considerable period of time. This is why the AA/EPA ratio in the blood is your ideal early-warning beacon that your wellness is eroding. The other trouble about CRP as a clinical marker of cellular inflammation is that very slight bacterial infections can cause it to become elevated. This makes it unreliable as a marker of chronic cellular inflammation. This is why if your CRP is elevated, it is usually recommended to retake the test in a few weeks to make sure it wasn't caused a slight bacterial infection.

If the AA/EPA ratio in the blood is the best marker of your ongoing ability to control cellular inflammation, then what should your levels be? After thousands of blood tests in Americans and data reported from Italians and Japanese, I can give you some guidelines:

AA/EPA Ratio	Comments	Reason
Less than 1.5	Too low	May increase bleeding
1.5–3	Ideal	Balanced inflammatory response
3–6	Good	
6–10	Needs work	Starting to reach a tipping point of increased cellular inflammation
10–15	Poor	Cellular inflammation is now widespread
Greater than 15	At risk	Chronic disease is probably developing

Ideally, you want to have your AA/EPA ratio between 1.5 and 3. As the AA/EPA ratio increases, so does your level of cellular inflammation. The average AA/EPA ratio in Americans is about 20. This is why American health care is crumbling—not from a lack of resources, but because Americans have a consistently and significantly high rate of cellular inflammation.

The fastest way to reduce the AA/EPA ratio is to take supplemental omega-3 fatty acids. The more you follow the Mediterranean Zone, the lower the levels of omega-3 fatty acids you will need since the Mediterranean Zone greatly restricts the intake of omega-6 fatty acids and moderates insulin levels that are both needed to produce AA. Adding supplemental omega-3 fatty acids will speed the process considerably so that within thirty days of following the Mediterranean Zone, you will begin to see a significant change in the AA/EPA ratio.

There are a number of private laboratories that do such AA/EPA testing. Some of these are listed below:

OmegaQuant (www.omegaquant.com)
MetaMatrix (www.metametrix.com)
Zone Diagnostics (www.zonediagnostics.com)

The prices range from $75 to $200 for the test. However, this may be the most important investment you can make in your future health.

Long-term Blood Sugar Control

The second marker of wellness is your level of glycosylated hemoglobin. Glucose is a very reactive compound that can link to proteins creating what is called advanced glycosylated endproducts (AGE). The formation of these AGE compounds comes from the Maillard reaction that occurs any time you have glucose, protein, and heat mixed together in a test tube. The same chemical reaction occurs inside your body if glucose levels become elevated in the blood. The resulting glycosylated proteins are sticky and end up in all the wrong places, such as the kidney, the eye, and the heart. Actually, it is even more complicated than that since there are receptors for these glycosylated proteins (known as RAGE) that if activated, initiate inflammatory responses through activation of NF-κB. RAGEs are similar to toll-like receptors in that they are based on pattern recognition. Although all proteins can become glycosylated in the presence of blood glucose, the most studied is glycosylated hemoglobin known as HbA_1c. Since hemoglobin is a long-lived protein, the levels of HbA_1c give an excellent marker of the long-term levels of glucose in the blood. The higher the HbA_1c levels, the more AGE products you have in the blood to interact with their receptors (RAGE), thus continually flaming cellular inflammation by activating NF-κB. To make matters worse, the more you activate NF-κB, the more RAGE receptors are synthesized. The result is a fast-forwarding of cellular inflammation. This is why the levels of RAGE are strongly associated with increased diabetes, heart disease, cancer, and Alzheimer's, all inflammatory diseases.

What are the levels of glycosylated hemoglobin that are consistent with longevity? These levels (expressed in percent of the total red blood cells) are shown below:

Ideal	Good	Poor	High Risk	Diabetic
5.0%	5.5%	6.0%	6.5%	> 7%

Shouldn't a lower percentage of glycosylated hemoglobin be even better? Not necessarily, since mortality begins to increase if glycosylated hemoglobin levels are too low. Low levels may indicate that the brain is not getting enough glucose to perform optimally. Like all markers of wellness, there is a zone.

The best way to reduce AGEs and RAGEs is simply not to consume a lot of carbohydrates, especially grains and starches, since they are composed of long polymers that are pure glucose. The best dietary solution to reduce AGE formation is to eat a lot of non-starchy vegetables The more non-starchy vegetables that you use as your carbohydrate source in your diet, the better the long-term blood sugar control. Since the lifetime of the red cells is 120 days, give yourself about four months to see a significant difference. Another dietary approach is to reduce the activation of NF-κB by consuming lots of polyphenols and omega-3 fatty acids. This is exactly what following the Mediterranean Zone accomplishes.

Insulin Resistance

The final marker of wellness is the degree of insulin resistance in your body. A primary function of insulin is to reduce blood glucose levels by driving glucose into its target cells. (The brain requires a lot of glucose, but it doesn't require insulin for the uptake of glucose into the brain.) Insulin resistance is caused by cellular inflammation interfering with the signaling that occurs when insulin binds to its receptor on the surface of the cell and disrupts the transmission of the signal into the cell. It's as if the insulin wasn't present in the first place.

The three major organs that are responsive to insulin interacting with its receptor are the adipose tissue, liver, and muscles (including heart muscles). Although the first place that insulin resistance starts is usually in your fat cells, the earliest clinical indication that insulin resistance is spreading is found in your liver.

The liver is the primary manufacturing site for taking in fats and re-packaging them in the form of lipoproteins for delivery to peripheral tissues. Insulin resistance disrupts this lipid repackaging process. Triglyceride levels rise, high-density cholesterol levels decrease, and low-density lipoproteins become smaller, more dense, and more atherogenic (more likely to increase the formation of plaques in the arteries). All of these risk factors increase the likelihood of developing cardiovascular disease. The reason that these small dense LDL particles are atherogenic is that it appears they are more easily oxidized in the blood. This is why the levels of oxidized LDL are far more predictive of future heart disease than total LDL levels are.

As insulin resistance (really cellular inflammation) spreads to the muscle, the glucose in the blood stays elevated, increasing the production of more glycosylated proteins (AGE) that increase inflammation throughout the body.

The best way to measure insulin resistance is by using a euglycemic insulin clamp, which is an extremely complex procedure done only under research conditions. The best surrogate marker of insulin resistance is the ratio of triglycerides (TG) to high-density lipoprotein (HDL) cholesterol in the blood. The higher the TG/HDL ratio, the greater the level of insulin resistance in the liver.

So what are good levels of the TG/HDL ratio? These are shown below:

Ideal	Fair	Poor	At risk
<1	1–2	3.5	>3.5

You usually find a TG/HDL ratio of less than one in elite athletes or people who follow the Mediterranean Zone. The average American has a TG/HDL ratio of 3.5, indicative of developing widespread insulin resistance. By the time the TG/HDL is greater than 4, you have metabolic syndrome (pre-diabetes) or fully developed type 2 diabetes.

An alternative method of determining insulin resistance is the levels of fasting insulin. This is a more expensive test than the TG/HDL ratio so insurance companies don't like to reimburse it. If you are able to get such a test, here are the numbers you are looking for in terms international units per ml (IU/ml).

Ideal	Fair	Poor	At risk
<5	5–10	10–15	>15

Since insulin resistance is the result of cellular inflammation, by following a strict Mediterranean Zone dietary program supplemented with purified omega-3 fatty acids and polyphenols, you can expect to see significant changes within thirty days.

Once you are in the Zone, your challenge is to stay there for a lifetime. These markers of wellness will provide continued clinical sentinels in the blood to alert you if you are moving out of the Zone. The correction to get back into the Zone is easy. Just follow the dietary instructions in this book.

Appendix G

Polyphenol Values

ow do you measure the levels of polyphenols in a food? The easiest indirect way is to determine the ORAC (oxygen radical absorption capacity) value. The technology to measure these values was developed in the 1990s to evaluate the anti-oxidant capacity of various foods. Although the ORAC value is related to the polyphenols found in a food, it doesn't totally distinguish between polyphenols and other anti-oxidants in a particular food. To be totally useful, ORAC values should be further refined to measure the levels of anti-oxidant potential relative to the levels of absorbable carbohydrate (total carbohydrates minus fiber) in a food. Whole grains have good ORAC levels, but very high levels of absorbable carbohydrate levels relative to fruits and vegetables. The extra carbohydrate will significantly impact insulin levels, reducing the benefits of the associated polyphenol in that food. Therefore the higher the ORAC/gram of absorbable carbohydrates, the greater the impact that food ingredient will have on reducing cellular inflammation.

ORAC values are only indicative of the anti-oxidant capacity in an artificial laboratory situation because it tells us nothing about the absorption or anti-oxidant actions in the blood. As an example, a study at Tufts Medical School indicated that doubling the ORAC intake of fruits and vegetables increased the levels of anti-oxidants in the blood by about 10 percent. This is why you have to consume a lot of polyphenol-containing foods to make an appreciable impact on the blood levels.

However, as I stated earlier in this book, the real purpose of polyphenols is to control the composition of the bacteria community in the gut. From that perspective, I believe that getting ten thousand ORAC units per day is a reasonable dietary goal to try to achieve to not only help control the bacteria in the gut, but also to improve the levels in the blood.

Listed below are the ORAC units for 100 grams of a variety of foods as well as the amount of total carbohydrates and fiber in each. Subtracting the fiber from the total carbohydrates gives us the carbohydrates available to enter the bloodstream and thus an indication of the food's impact on insulin secretion. The goal of the Mediterranean Zone is to use primarily the foods that have the most polyphenols with the least amount of available carbohydrates.

FRUITS

Fruits	ORAC Units/100 g	Calories/ 100 g	Grams Absorbable Carbs/100 g	ORAC Units/gram of Absorbable Carbs
Apples, raw, with skin	3,049	52	11	282
Apricots, raw	1,110	48	9	122
Avocados, raw	1,371	160	2	749
Bananas, raw	795	89	20	39
Blackberries, raw	5,905	43	4	1,370
Blueberries, raw	4,669	57	12	386
Blueberries, wild, raw	9,621	61	10	991
Cherries, sweet, raw	3,747	63	14	269
Cranberries, raw	9,090	46	8	1,196
Currants, black, raw	7,957	63	15	517
Dates, un-cooked	3,895	282	67	58
Elderberries, raw	14,697	73	11	1,289
Figs, raw	3,383	47	16	208
Grapefruit, raw, pink and red	1,548	42	9	171
Grapes, red, raw	1,837	69	17	107
Guavas, raw	1,422	68	9	159
Kiwi, raw	862	61	12	74
Lemons, raw, without peel	1,346	29	7	206
Lime juice, raw	823	25	8	103
Limes, raw	82	30	8	11
Mangos, raw	1,300	60	13	97

Fruits	ORAC Units/100 g	Calories/ 100 g	Grams Absorbable Carbs/100 g	ORAC Units/gram of Absorbable Carbs
Melons, canta-loupe, raw	319	34	7	44
Melons, honey-dew, raw	253	36	8	31
Nectarines, raw	919	44	9	104
Oranges, raw	2,103	47	9	225
Papayas, raw	300	43	9	33
Peaches, canned, heavy syrup, drained	436	72	17	25
Peaches, raw	1,922	39	8	239
Pears, raw	1,746	57	12	142
Pineapple, raw, all varieties	385	50	11	33
Plums, raw	6,100	46	10	609
Pomegranates, raw	4,479	83	15	305
Prunes, un-cooked	8,059	240	57	142
Raisins, golden seedless	10,450	302	76	138
Raisins, seed-less	3,406	299	75	45
Raspberries, raw	5,065	52	5	931
Strawberries, raw	4,302	32	6	757
Tangerines, raw	1,627	53	12	141
Watermelon, raw	142	30	7	20

VEGETABLES

Vegetables	ORAC Units/100 g	Calories/ 100 g	Grams Absorbable Carbs/100 g	ORAC Units/gram of Absorbable Carbs
Artichokes (globe), raw	6,552	47	5	1,282
Arugula, raw	1,904	25	2	929
Asparagus, cooked, boiled, drained	1,644	22	2	779
Asparagus, raw	2,252	20	2	1,265
Asparagus, white, raw	296	20	2	166
Beans, snap, green, raw	799	31	4	187
Beets, raw	1,776	43	7	263
Broccoli, raw	1,510	34	4	356
Cabbage, raw	529	25	3	160
Cabbage, red, raw	2,496	31	5	474
Carrots, raw	697	41	7	103
Catsup	578	112	26	22
Cauliflower, raw	870	25	3	293
Celery, raw	552	16	1	403
Chives, raw	2,094	30	2	1,132
Coriander (cilantro) leaves, raw	5,141	23	1	5,909
Corn, sweet, yellow, frozen	522	88	19	28
Corn, sweet, yellow, raw	728	86	17	44
Cucumber, peeled, raw	140	12	1	96

Vegetables	ORAC Units/100 g	Calories/ 100 g	Grams Absorbable Carbs/100 g	ORAC Units/gram of Absorbable Carbs
Cucumber, with peel, raw	232	15	3	74
Eggplant, boiled	245	33	6	43
Eggplant, raw	932	25	3	324
Fennel, bulb, raw	307	31	4	73
Garlic, raw	5,708	149	21	184
Ginger root, raw	14,840	80	16	941
Leeks (bulb and lower leaf-portion), raw	569	61	12	46
Lettuce, romaine, raw	1,017	17	1	855
Lettuce, iceberg, raw	438	14	2	247
Lettuce, red leaf, raw	2,426	16	1	1,784
Mushrooms, oyster, raw	664	33	4	175
Mushrooms, portobello, raw	968	22	3	377
Mushrooms, white, raw	691	22	2	306
Onions, raw	913	40	8	120
Onions, sweet, raw	614	32	7	92
Parsley, raw	1,220	36	3	403
Peas, green, frozen, unprepared	600	77	9	66
Peppers, sweet, green, raw	935	20	3	318

Vegetables	ORAC Units/100 g	Calories/ 100 g	Grams Absorbable Carbs/100 g	ORAC Units/gram of Absorbable Carbs
Peppers, sweet, red, raw	821	31	4	209
Peppers, sweet, yellow, raw	1,043	27	5	192
Potatoes, red, flesh and skin, raw	1,098	70	14	77
Potatoes, russet, flesh and skin, raw	1,322	70	14	93
Potatoes, white, flesh and skin, raw	1,058	69	13	79
Pumpkin, raw	483	26	6	81
Radishes, raw	1,750	16	2	972
Spinach, raw	1,513	23	1	1,058
Squash, summer, zucchini, includes skin, raw	180	17	2	85
Squash, winter, butternut, raw	396	45	10	41
Sweet potato, raw	902	86	17	53
Tomatoes, red, ripe, raw, year-round average	387	18	3	144

BREAKFAST CEREALS

Breakfast Cereals	ORAC Units/100 g	Calories/ 100 g	Grams Absorbable Carbs/100 g	ORAC Units/gram of Absorbable Carbs
Cereals ready-to-eat, oatmeal	1,517	374	71	21
Cereals, corn flakes	2,359	399	87	27
Cereals, shred-ded wheat	1,303	337	67	20

OILS AND NUTS

Oils and Nuts	ORAC Units/100 g	Calories/ 100 g	Grams Absorbable Carbs/100 g	ORAC Units/gram of Absorbable Carbs
Oil, peanut, salad or cooking	106	884	n/a	n/a
Olive oil, extra-virgin	372	880	n/a	n/a

LEGUMES

Legumes	ORAC Units/100 g	Calories/ 100 g	Grams Absorbable Carbs/100 g	ORAC Units/gram of Absorbable Carbs
Beans, black, mature seeds, raw	8,494	341	47	181

Legumes	ORAC Units/100 g	Calories/ 100 g	Grams Absorbable Carbs/100 g	ORAC Units/gram of Absorbable Carbs
Beans, kidney, red, mature seeds, raw	8,606	337	46	187
Beans, navy, mature seeds, raw	1,861	337	36	51
Beans, pink, mature seeds, raw	8,320	343	51	162
Beans, pinto, mature seeds, boiled	904	143	17	19
Beans, pinto, mature seeds, raw	8,033	347	47	171
Black-eyed peas, raw	4,343	336	49	88
Chickpeas (garbanzo beans), raw	847	364	43	20
Lentils, raw	7,282	353	29	246
Peanut butter, smooth style	3,432	588	13	253
Peanuts, all types, raw	3,166	567	7	415
Peas, split, mature seeds, raw	524	341	35	15
Peas, yellow, mature seeds, raw	741	345	36	21
Soybeans, mature seeds, raw	5,409	446	21	259

BREADS

Breads	ORAC Units/100 g	Calories/ 100 g	Grams Absorbable Carbs/100 g	ORAC Units/gram of Absorbable Carbs
Bread, pumpernickel	1,963	250	41	48
Bread, wholegrain	1,421	265	36	40

BEVERAGES

Beverages	ORAC Units/100 g	Calories/ 100 g	Grams Absorbable Carbs/100 g	ORAC Units/gram of Absorbable Carbs
Alcoholic beverage, wine, table, red	3,607	85	3	1,382
Alcoholic Beverage, wine, table, red, Cabernet Sauvignon	4,523	83	3	1,740
Alcoholic Beverage, wine, table, red, Merlot	2,670	83	3	1,064
Alcoholic Beverage, wine, table, red, Zinfandel	2,400	88	3	839

Beverages	ORAC Units/100 g	Calories/ 100 g	Grams Absorbable Carbs/100 g	ORAC Units/gram of Absorbable Carbs
Alcoholic beverage, wine, table, white	392	82	3	151
Tea, brewed, prepared with tap water	1,128	1	0	3,760

SPICES AND HERBS

Spices & Herbs	ORAC Units/100 g	Calories/ 100 g	Grams Absorbable Carbs/100 g	ORAC Units/gram of Absorbable Carbs
Basil, fresh	4,805	23	1	4,576
Basil, dried	61,063	23	10	6,076
Chili powder	23,636	282	15	1,586
Cinnamon, ground	13,142	247	28	478
Cloves, ground	29,028	274	32	918
Cumin seed	50,372	375	34	1,493
Curry powder	48,504	325	25	1,944
Dill weed, fresh	4,392	43	5	893
Garlic powder	6,665	331	64	105
Ginger, ground	39,041	335	58	679
Mustard seed, yellow	29,257	508	16	1,841
Nutmeg, ground	69,640	525	29	2,444
Onion powder	4,289	341	64	67
Oregano, dried	175,295	265	26	6,635
Paprika	21,932	282	19	1,149
Parsley, dried	73,670	292	24	3,077
Pepper, black	34,053	251	39	881

Spices & Herbs	ORAC Units/100 g	Calories/ 100 g	Grams Absorbable Carbs/100 g	ORAC Units/gram of Absorbable Carbs
Pepper, red or cayenne	19,671	318	30	668
Pepper, white	40,700	296	42	960
Peppermint, fresh	13,978	70	7	2,029
Rosemary, dried	165,280	331	21	7,702
Sage, ground	119,929	315	20	5,870
Thyme, dried	157,380	276	27	5,842
Turmeric, ground	127,068	354	44	2,899
Vinegar, Apple	564	21	1	606
Vinegar, Red wine	410	19	0	1,519

SWEETS AND SNACKS

Sweets	ORAC Units/100 g	Calories/ 100 g	Grams Absorbable Carbs/100 g	ORAC Units/gram of Absorbable Carbs
Agave, raw (Southwest)	1,294	68	10	134
Baking choco-late, unsweet-ened, squares	49,944	501	13	3,772
Candies, milk chocolate	7,519	535	56	134
Candies, semi-sweet chocolate	18,053	480	58	311

Sweets	ORAC Units/100 g	Calories/ 100 g	Grams Absorbable Carbs/100 g	ORAC Units/gram of Absorbable Carbs
Cocoa, dry powder, unsweetened	55,653	228	25	2,253
Syrups, maple	590	260	67	9
Snacks	ORAC Units/100 g	Calories/ 100 g	Grams Absorbable Carbs/100 g	ORAC Units/gram of Absorbable Carbs
Snacks, popcorn, air popped	1,743	387	63	27

A number of things become apparent once you look at these charts. First, herbs and spices have the greatest amount of ORAC units per gram of carbohydrate. This is why their primary purpose in the Mediterranean Zone is to provide anti-oxidants, not just flavor. Second, vegetables have a wide range of ORAC units/gram of carbohydrate. When you overcook vegetables, as you do when you boil them until they become limp and gray, you destroy much of their polyphenol content. Third, some fruits, such as berries, are excellent sources of polyphenols with the least amount of carbohydrates. Others, such as watermelon, are not. Fourth, the polyphenols in whole grains come with an exceedingly high carbohydrate content. Fifth, red wines are rich in polyphenols, but so is tea. Finally, relatively unprocessed dark chocolate is a great source of polyphenols, but the commercial products made from them are far less desirable. This is because the processing (alkali refining) used to make most commercial dark chocolates as well as candy bars destroys most of the polyphenols.

Although ORAC measurements are the easiest way to estimate polyphenol levels, the best way to directly analyze their content is by more sophisticated techniques such as high-pressure liquid chromatography. When possible, I have compared these numbers to the ORAC levels of the same foods. The results of such polyphenol analysis of common food ingredients are shown below.

Food ingredient	Polyphenols (mg/100 g or 100 ml)	ORAC (100 g)
Purified polyphenol extracts		
Delphinol® (maqui berry)	35,200	2,835,280
Herbs and Spices		
Oregano, dried	2,137	175,295
Sage, dried	893	119,929
Rosemary, dried	522	165,280
Thyme, dried	464	157,380
Curry powder	285	48,504
Ginger, dried	202	39,041
Basil, dried	166	61,063
Cumin	55	50,372
Chocolate		
Cocoa powder	3,294	55,683
Dark chocolate	1,618	18,053
Milk chocolate	236	7,519
Fruits		
Elderberry	804	14,697
Blueberry	496	9,631
Caper	389	unknown
Black olive	320	unknown
Plum	285	6,100
Strawberry	205	4,302
Blackberry	180	5,905
Cherry	145	3,747
Apple	136	3,049
Raspberry	107	5,065
Peach	54	1,922
Nectarine	20	919
Apricot	15	1,100
Pear	11	1,746

Food ingredient	Polyphenols (mg/100 g or 100 ml)	ORAC (100 g)
Vegetables		
Artichoke head	154	6,552
Red onion	99	913
Spinach	68	1,513
Broccoli	21	1,510
Red lettuce	14	2,426
Asparagus	11	1,644
Carrot	7	697
Legumes		
Soybean	153	5,409
Black bean	36	8,494
White bean	31	unknown
Tofu	25	unknown
Whole Grain Flours		
Flaxseed	1,220	unknown
Rye	143	unknown
Wheat	71	unknown
Oat	37	unknown
Nuts and Oils		
Chestnut	1,215	unknown
Pecan	493	unknown
Almond	185	unknown
Extra-virgin olive oil	33	372
Walnut	28	unknown
Beverages		
Coffee, filtered	105	unknown
Red wine	91	3,607
Green tea	82	1,128
White wine	9	392

Although there is a correlation between ORAC values and polyphenol levels, there is also great variability. This is because ORAC values are measuring both polyphenols and non-polyphenol anti-oxidants. The richest food source of polyphenols is cocoa powder. Although cocoa is really a fruit, I put it into a separate category as chocolate. Cocoa power is not only among one of the best sources of polyphenols but also one of the most user-friendly food ingredients. But the "best of the best" for polyphenol content appears to be the highly purified extract from the maqui berry, which contains 25 percent by weight of delphinidins. It is the only purified polyphenol (known by the trade name Delphinol) that also has GRAS status as a food additive. Adding Delphinol to cocoa powder gives you "super chocolate" that is great way for making healthy chocolate desserts ideally suited for the Mediterranean Zone.

Appendix H

References

INTRODUCTION

Agus MS, Swain JF, Larson CL, Eckert EA, and Ludwig DS. "Dietary composition and physiologic adaptations to energy restriction." Am J Clin Nutr 71: 901–907 (2000)

Dumesnil JG, Turgeon J, Tremblay A, Poirier P, Gilbert M, Gagnon L, St-Pierre S, Garneau C, Lemieux I, Pascot A, Bergeron J, and Despres JP. "Effect of a low-glycaemic index—low-fat—high protein diet on the atherogenic metabolic risk profile of abdominally obese men." Br J Nutr 86: 557–568 (2001)

Ebbeling CB, Leidig MM, Feldman HA, Lovesky MM, and Ludwig DS. "Effects of a low-glycemic load vs low-fat diet in obese young adults: a randomized trial." JAMA 297: 2092–2102 (2007)

Gannon MC and Nuttall FQ. "Control of blood glucose in type 2 diabetes without weight loss by modification of diet composition." Nutr Metab 3: 16 (2006)

Hamdy O and Carver C. "The Why WAIT program: improving clinical outcomes through weight management in type 2 diabetes." Curr Diab Rep 8: 413–420 (2008)

Johnston CS, Tjonn SL, Swan PD, White A, Hutchins H, and Sears B. "Ketogenic low-carbohydrate diets have no metabolic advantage over nonketogenic low-carbohydrate diets." Am J Clin Nutr 83: 1055–1061 (2006)

Lasker DA, Evans EM, and Layman DK. "Moderate carbohydrate, moderate protein weight loss diet reduces cardiovascular disease risk compared to high carbohydrate, low protein diet in obese adults: A randomized clinical trial." Nutr Metab 5: 30 (2008)

Layman DK, Boileau RA, Erickson DJ, Painter JE, Shiue H, Sather C, and Christou DD. "A reduced ratio of dietary carbohydrate to protein improves body composition and blood lipid profiles during weight loss in adult women." J Nutr 133: 411–417 (2003)

Layman DK, Shiue H, Sather C, Erickson DJ, and Baum J. "Increased dietary protein modifies glucose and insulin homeostasis in adult women during weight loss." J Nutr 133: 405–410 (2003)

Layman DK, Evans EM, Erickson D, Seyler J, Weber J, Bagshaw D, Griel A, Psota T, and Kris-Etherton P. "A moderate-protein diet produces sustained weight loss and long-term changes in body composition and blood lipids in obese adults." J Nutr 139: 514–521 (2009)

Ludwig DS, Majzoub JA, Al-Zahrani A, Dallal GE, Blanco I, and Roberts SB. "High glycemic index foods, overeating, and obesity." Pediatrics 103: E26 (1999)

Markovic TP, Campbell LV, Balasubramanian S, Jenkins AB, Fleury AC, Simons LA, and Chisholm DJ. "Beneficial effect on average lipid levels from energy restriction and fat loss in obese individuals with or without type 2 diabetes." Diabetes Care 21: 695–700 (1998)

Nuttall FQ, Gannon MC, Saeed A, Jordan K, and Hoover H. "The metabolic response of subjects with type 2 diabetes to a high-protein, weight-maintenance diet." J Clin Endocrinol Metab 2003 88: 3577–3583 (2003)

Oates JA. "The 1982 Nobel Prize in Physiology or Medicine." Science 218: 765–768 (1982)

Pereira MA, Swain J, Goldfine AB, Rifai N, and Ludwig DS. "Effects of a low-glycemic load diet on resting energy expenditure and heart disease risk factors during weight loss." JAMA 292: 2482–2490 (2004)

Sears B. *The Zone*. Regan Books. New York, NY (1995)

Sears B. *The OmegaRx Zone*. Regan Books. New York, NY (2002)

Tollefsbol T (ed). *Epigenetics in Human Disease*. Academic Press. New York, NY (2012)

CHAPTER 1: THE COMING RECKONING

Alzheimer's Organization. 2013 Alzheimer's Disease Facts and Figures. (2013)

Crane PK, Walker R, Hubbard RA, Li G, Nathan DM, Zheng H, Haneuse S, Craft S, Montine TJ, Kahn SE, McCormick W, McCurry SM, Bowen JD, and Larson EB. "Glucose levels and risk of dementia." N Engl J Med 369: 540–548 (2013)

James BD, Leurgans SE, Hebert LE, Scherr PA, Yaffe K, and Bennett DA. "Contribution of Alzheimer disease to mortality in the United States." Neurology 82: 1045–1050 (2014)

Holmes C. "Review: systemic inflammation and Alzheimer's disease." Neuropathol Appl Neurobiol 39: 51–68 (2013)

Mehla J, Chauhan BC, and Chauhan NB. "Experimental induction of type 2 diabetes in aging-accelerated mice triggered Alzheimer-like pathology and memory deficits." J Alzheimer's Dis 39: 145–162 (2014)

Ohara T, Doi Y, Ninomiya T, Hirakawa Y, Hata J, Iwaki T, Kanba S, and Kiyohara Y. "Glucose tolerance status and risk of dementia in the community: the Hisayama study." Neurology 77: 1126–1134 (2011)

Sears B. *The Zone*. Regan Books. New York, NY (1995)

Spite M, Claria J, and Serhan CN. "Resolvins, specialized proresolving lipid mediators and their potential roles in metabolic diseases." Cell Metabolism 19: 21–36 (2014)

Wang X , Zhu M, Hjorth E, Cortés-Toro V, Eyjolfsdottir H, Graff C, Nennesmo I, Palmblad J, Eriksdotter M , Sambamurti K, Fitzgerald JM , Serhan CN , Granholm AC, and Schultzberg M. "Resolution of inflammation is altered in Alzheimer's disease." Alzheimers Dement 10: doi: 10.1016/j.jalz.2013.12.024 (2014)

CHAPTER 2: INFLAMMATION: THE REAL REASON WE GAIN WEIGHT, GET SICK, AND AGE FASTER

Alzheimer's Organization. 2013 Alzheimer's Disease Facts and Figures. (2013)

Berg JM, Tymoczko JL, and Stryer L. *Biochemistry, 5th edition.* W.H. Freeman. New York, NY (2002)

Blasbalg TL, Hibbeln JR, Ramsden CE, Majchrzak SF, and Rawlings RR. "Changes in consumption of omega-3 and omega-6 fatty acids in the United States during the 20th century." Am J Clin Nutr 93: 950–962 (2011)

Centers for Disease Control. www.cdc.gov/aging/aginginfo/alzheimers.htm (2011)

Czech MP, Tencerova M, Pedersen DJ, and Aouadi M. "Insulin signaling mechanisms for triacylglycerol storage." Diabetologia 56: 949–964 (2013)

Dimitriadis G, Mitrou P, Lambadiari V, Maratou E, and Raptis SA. "Insulin effects in muscle and adipose tissue." Diabetes Res Clin Pract 93: S52–59 (2011)

Liebman B. "The changing American diet." Nutritional Action Newsletter. September, 2013 (http: //cspinet.org/new/pdf/changing_american_diet_13.pdf) (2013)

Nam TG. "Lipid peroxidation and its toxicological implications." Toxicol Res 27: 1–6 (2011)

Ohara T, Doi Y, Ninomiya T, Hirakawa Y, Hata J, Iwaki T, Kanba S, and Kiyohara Y. "Glucose tolerance status and risk of dementia in the community: the Hisayama study." Neurology 77: 1126–1134 (2011)

Sadur CN and Eckel RH. "Insulin stimulation of adipose tissue lipoprotein Lipase" J Clin. Invest 69: 1119–1123 (1982)

Scalbert A, Johnson IT, and Saltmarsh M. "Polyphenols: antioxidants and beyond." Am J Clin Nutr 81: 215S–217S (2005)

Schenk S, Saberi M, and Olefsky JM. "Insulin sensitivity: modulation by nutrients and inflammation." J Clin Invest 118: 2992–3002 (2008)

Sears B. *The Zone.* Regan Books. New York, NY (1995)

Sears B. *The Anti-Aging Zone.* Regan Books. New York, NY (1999)

Sears B. *The Anti-Inflammation Zone.* Regan Books. New York, NY (2005)

Sears B. *Toxic Fat.* Thomas Nelson. Nashville, TN (2008)

Tabues G. "Prosperity's Plague." Science 325: 256–260 (2009)

Xu A, Wang Y, Xu JY, Stejskal D, Tam S, Zhang J, Wat NM, Wong WK, and Lam KS. "Adipocyte fatty acid-binding protein is a plasma biomarker closely associated with obesity and metabolic syndrome." Clin Chem 52: 405–413 (2006)

CHAPTER 3. THE ZONE DIET: ANTI-INFLAMMATORY NUTRITION MADE SIMPLE

Bell SJ and Sears B. "Low-glycemic-load diets: impact on obesity and chronic diseases." Crit Rev Food Sci Nutr 43: 357–377 (2003)

Berg JM, Tymoczko JL, and Stryer L. *Biochemistry, 5th edition.* W.H. Freeman. New York, NY (2002)

Bierhaus A, Stern DM, and Nawroth PP. "RAGE in inflammation: a new therapeutic target?"Curr Opin Investig Drugs 7: 985–991 (2006)

Curtiss LK. "Reversing atherosclerosis?" N Engl J Med 360: 1144–1146 (2009)

Davidenko O, Darcel N, Fromentin G, and Tome D. "Control of protein and energy intake - brain mechanisms." Eur J Clin Nutr 67: 455–461 (2013)

Ebbeling CB, Swain JF, Feldman HA, Wong WW, Hachey DL, Garcia-Lago E, and Ludwig DS. "Effects of dietary composition on energy expenditure during weight-loss maintenance." JAMA 307: 2627–2634 (2012)

Holvoet P. "Oxidized LDL and coronary heart disease." Acta Cardiol 59: 479–484 (2004)

Ishigaki Y, Oka Y, and Katagiri H. "Circulating oxidized LDL: a biomarker and a pathogenic factor." Curr Opin Lipidol 20: 363–369 (2009)

Johnston CS, Tjonn SL, Swan PD, White A, Hutchins H, and Sears B. "Ketogenic low-carbohydrate diets have no metabolic advantage over nonketogenic low-carbohydrate diets." Am J Clin Nutr 83: 1055–1061 (2006)

Joslin Diabetes Research Center. www.joslin.org/docs/Nutrition_Guideline_Graded.pdfEPIC and Diabetes (2007)

Kawabata T, Hirota S, Hirayama T, Adachi N, Hagiwara C, Iwama N, Kamachi K, Araki E, Kawashima H, and Kiso Y. "Age-related changes of dietary intake and blood eicosapentaenoic acid, docosahexaenoic acid, and arachidonic acid levels in Japanese men and women." Prostaglandins Leukot Essent Fatty Acids 84: 131–137 (2011)

Kuipers RS, Luxwolda MF, Dijck-Brouwer DA, Eaton SB, Crawford MA, Cordain L, and Muskiet FA. "Estimated macronutrient and fatty acid intakes from an East African Paleolithic diet." Br J Nutr 104: 1666–1687 (2010)

Ludwig DS, Majzoub JA, Al-Zahrani A, Dallal GE, Blanco I, and Roberts SB. "High glycemic index foods, overeating, and obesity." Pediatrics 103: E26 (1999)

McLaughlin T, Reaven G, Abbasi F, Lamendola C, Saad M, Waters D, Simon J, and Krauss RM. "Is there a simple way to identify insulin-resistant individuals at increased risk of cardiovascular disease?" Am J Cardiol 96: 399–404 (2005)

Pereira MA, Swain J, Goldfine AB, Rifai N, and Ludwig DS. "Effects of a low-glycemic load diet on resting energy expenditure and heart disease risk factors during weight loss." JAMA 292: 2482–2490 (2004)

Pittas AG, Roberts SB, Das SK, Gilhooly CH, Saltzman E, Golden J, Stark PC, and Greenberg AS. "The effects of the dietary glycemic load on type 2 diabetes risk factors during weight loss." Obesity 14: 2200–2209 (2006)

Ramasamy R, Vannucci SJ, Yan SS, Herold K, Yan SF, and Schmidt AM. "Advanced glycation end products and RAGE: a common thread in aging, diabetes, neurodegeneration, and inflammation." Glycobiology 15: 16R–28R (2005)

Sears B. *The Zone.* Regan Books. New York, NY (1995)

Sears B. *Mastering the Zone.* Regan Books. New York, NY (1997)

Sears B. *Zone Perfect Meals in Minutes.* Regan Books. New York, NY (1998)

Sears B. *The OmegaRx Zone.* Regan Books. New York, NY (2002)

Sears B and Sears L. *Zone Meals in Seconds.* Regan Books. New York, NY (2005)

Stout RL, Fulks M, Dolan VF, Magee ME, and Suarez L. "Relationship of hemoglobin A1c to mortality in nonsmoking insurance applicants." J Insur Med 39: 174–181 (2007)

Yokoyama M, Origasa H, Matsuzaki M, Matsuzawa Y, Saito Y, Ishikawa Y, Oikawa S, Sasaki J, Hishida H, Itakura H, Kita T, Kitabatake A, Nakaya N, Sakata T, Shimada K. and Shirato K. "Effects of eicosapentaenoic acid on major coronary events in hypercholesterolaemic patients (JELIS): a randomised open-label, blinded endpoint analysis." Lancet 369: 1090–1098 (2007)

CHAPTER 4: FACTS AND FICTION ABOUT THE MEDITERRANEAN DIET

Ahrens EH. "Dietary fats and coronary heart disease: unfinished business." Lancet 2: 1345–1348 (1979)

American Heart Association. "Dietary guidelines for healthy American adults. A statement for physicians and health professionals by the Nutrition Committee, American Heart Association." Circulation 77: 721–724A (1988)

Boccardi V, Esposito A, Rizzo MR, Marfella R, Barbieri M, and Paolisso G. "Mediterranean diet, telomere maintenance and health status among elderly." PLoS ONE 8: e62781 (2013)

Buckland G, Bach A, and Serra-Majem L. "Obesity and the Mediterranean diet: a systematic review of observational and intervention studies." Obes 9: 582–593 (2008)

Buckland G, Agudo A, Travier N, Huerta JM, Cirera L, Tormo MJ, Navarro C, Chirlaque MD, Moreno-Iribas C, Ardanaz E, Barricarte A, Etxeberria J, Marin P, Quirós JR, Redondo ML, Larrañaga N, Amiano P, Dorronsoro M, Arriola L, Basterretxea M, Sanchez MJ, Molina E, and González CA. "Adherence to the Mediterranean diet reduces mortality in the Spanish cohort of the European Prospective Investigation into Cancer and Nutrition (EPIC-Spain)." Br J Nutr 106: 1581–1591 (2011)

Dedoussis GV, Kanoni S, Mariani E, Cattini L, Herbein G, Fulop T, Varin A, Rink L, Jajte J, Monti D, Marcellini F, Malavolta M, and Mocchegiani E. "Mediterranean diet and plasma concentration of inflammatory markers in old and very old subjects in the ZINCAGE population study." Clin Chem Lab Med 46: 990–996 (2008)

de Lorgeril M, Renaud S, Mamelle N, Salen P, Martin JL, Monjaud I, Guidollet J, Touboul P, and Delaye J. "Mediterranean alpha-linolenic acid-rich diet in secondary prevention of coronary heart disease." Lancet 343: 1454–1559 (1994)

de Lorgeril M, Salen P, Martin JL, Monjaud I, Boucher P, and Mamelle N. "Mediterranean dietary pattern in a randomized trial: prolonged survival and possible reduced cancer rate." Arch Intern Med 158: 1181–1187 (1998)

de Lorgeril M, Salen P, Martin JL, Monjaud I, Delaye J, and Mamelle N. "Mediterranean diet, traditional risk factors, and the rate of cardiovascular complications after myocardial infarction: final report of the Lyon Diet Heart Study." Circulation 99: 779–785 (1999)

de Lorgeril M and Salen P. "Mediterranean diet in secondary prevention of CHD." Public Health Nutr 14: 2333–2337 (2011)

de Lorgeril M. "Mediterranean diet and cardiovascular disease: historical perspective and latest evidence." Curr Athosclero Rep 15: 370 (2013)

Djuric Z. "The Mediterranean diet: effects on proteins that mediate fatty acid metabolism in the colon." Nutr Rev 69: 730–744 (2011)

Estruch R, Ros E, Salas-Salvadó J, Covas MI, Corella D, Arós F, Gómez-Gracia E, Ruiz-Gutiérrez V, Fiol M, Lapetra J, Lamuela-Raventos RM, Serra-Majem L, Pintó X, Basora J, Muñoz MA, Sorlí JV, Martínez JA, and Martínez-González MA. "Primary prevention of cardiovascular disease with a Mediterranean diet." N Engl J Med 368: 1279–1290 (2013)

Feart C, Samieri C, Rondeau V, Amieva H, Portet F, Dartigues JF, Scarmeas N, and Barberger-Gateau P. "Adherence to a Mediterranean diet, cognitive decline, and risk of dementia." JAMA 302: 638–648 (2009)

Feart C, Samieri C, and Barberger-Gateau P. "Mediterranean diet and cognitive function in older adults." Curr Opin Clin Nutr Metab Care 13: 14–18 (2010)

Feart C, Torres MJ, Samieri C, Jutand MA, Peuchant E, Simopoulos AP, and Barberger-Gateau P. "Adherence to a Mediterranean diet and plasma fatty acids: data from the Bordeaux sample of the Three-City study." Br J Nutr 106: 149–158 (2011)

Feart C, Torres MJ, Samieri C, Jutand MA, Peuchant E, Simopoulos AP, and Barberger-Gateau P. "Potential benefits of adherence to the Mediterranean diet on cognitive health." Proc Nutr Soc 72: 140–152 (2013)

Fragopoulou E, Panagiotakos DB, Pitsavos C, Tampourlou M, Chrysohoou C, Nomikos T, Antonopoulou S, and Stefanadis C. "The association between adherence to the Mediterranean diet and adiponectin levels among healthy adults: the ATTICA study." J Nutr Biochem 21: 285–289 (2010)

Gardener S, Gu Y, Rainey-Smith SR, Keogh JB, Clifton PM, Mathieson SL, Taddei K, Mondal A, Ward VK, Scarmeas N, Barnes M, Ellis KA, Head R, Masters CL, Ames D, Macaulay SL, Rowe CC, Szoeke C, and Martins RN. "Adherence to a Mediterranean diet and Alzheimer's disease risk in an Australian population." Transl Psychiatry 2: e164 (2012)

Hoevenaar-Blom MP, Nooyens AC, Kromhout D, Spijkerman AM, Beulens JW, van der Schouw YT, Bueno-de-Mesquita B, and Verschuren WM. "Mediterranean style diet and 12-year incidence of cardiovascular diseases: the EPIC-NL cohort study." PLoS ONE 7: e45458 (2012)

Itsiopoulos C, Brazionis L, Kaimakamis M, Cameron M, Best JD, O'Dea K, Rowley K. "Can the Mediterranean diet lower HbA1c in type 2 diabetes? Results from a randomized cross-over study." Nutr Metab Cardiovasc Dis 21: 740–747 (2011)

Jones JL, Comperatore M, Barona J, Calle MC, Andersen C, McIntosh M, Najm W, Lerman RH, and Fernandez ML. "A Mediterranean-style, low-glycemic-load diet decreases atherogenic lipoproteins and reduces lipoprotein (a) and oxidized low-density lipoprotein in women with metabolic syndrome." Metabolism 61: 366–372 (2012)

Kafatos A, Diacatou A, Voukiklaris G, Nikolakakis N, Vlachonikolis J, Kounali D, Mamalakis G, Dontas AS. "Heart disease risk-factor status and dietary changes in the Cretan population over the past 30 y: the Seven Countries Study." Am J Clin Nutr 65: 1882–1886 (1997)

Kesse-Guyot E, Andreeva VA, Lassale C, Ferry M, Jeandel C, Hercberg S, and Galan P. "Mediterranean diet and cognitive function: a French study." Am J Clin Nutr 97: 369–376 (2013)

Lourida I, Soni M, Thompson-Coon J, Purandare N, Lang IA, Ukoumunne OC, and Llewellyn DJ. "Mediterranean diet, cognitive function, and dementia: a systematic review." Epidemiology 24: 479–489 (2013)

Martínez-González MA, de la Fuente-Arrillaga C, Nunez-Cordoba JM, Basterra-

Gortari FJ, Beunza JJ, Vazquez Z, Benito S, Tortosa A, and Bes-Rastrollo M. "Adherence to Mediterranean diet and risk of developing diabetes: prospective cohort study." BMJ 336: 1348–1351 (2008)

Menotti A, Keys A, Kromhout D, Blackburn H, Aravanis C, Bloemberg B, Buzina R, Dontas A, Fidanza F, and Giampaoli S. "Inter-cohort differences in coronary heart disease mortality in the 25-year follow-up of the seven countries study." Eur J Epidemiol 9: 527–536 (1993)

Mitrou PN, Kipnis V, Thiébaut AC, Reedy J, Subar AF, Wirfält E, Flood A, Mouw T, Hollenbeck AR, Leitzmann MF, and Schatzkin A. "Mediterranean dietary pattern and prediction of all-cause mortality in a US population: results from the NIH-AARP Diet and Health Study." Arch Intern Med 167: 2461–2468 (2007)

Pitsavos C, Panagiotakos DB, Tzima N, Chrysohoou C, Economou M, Zampelas A, and Stefanadis C. "Adherence to the Mediterranean diet is associated with total antioxidant capacity in healthy adults: the ATTICA study." Am J Clin Nutr 82: 694–699 (2005)

Perez-Lopez FR, Chedraui P, Haya J, and Cuadros JL. "Effects of the Mediterranean diet on longevity and age-related morbid conditions." Maturitas 64: 67–79 (2009)

Salas-Salvadó J, Bulló M, Babio N, Martínez-González MÁ, Ibarrola-Jurado N, Basora J, Estruch R, Covas MI, Corella D, Arós F, Ruiz-Gutiérrez V, and Ros E. "Reduction in the incidence of type 2 diabetes with the Mediterranean diet: results of the PREDIMED-Reus nutrition intervention randomized trial." Diabetes Care 34: 14–19 (2011)

Renaud S and de Lorgeril M. "Wine, alcohol, platelets, and the French paradox for coronary heart disease." Lancet 339: 1523–1526 (1992)

Rossi M, Turati F, Lagiou P, Trichopoulos D, Augustin LS, La Vecchia C, and Trichopoulu. "Mediterranean diet and glycaemic load in relation to incidence of type 2 diabetes." Diabetologia 56: 2405–13 (2013)

Samieri C, Okereke OI, E Devore E, and Grodstein F. "Long-term adherence to the Mediterranean diet is associated with overall cognitive status, but not cognitive decline, in women." J Nutr 143: 493–499 (2013)

Samieri C, Grodstein F, Rosner BA, Kang JH, Cook NR, Manson JE, Buring JE, Willett WC, and Okereke OI. "Mediterranean diet and cognitive function in older age." Epidemiology 24: 490–499 (2013)

Scarmeas N, Luchsinger JA, Mayeux R, and Stern Y. "Mediterranean diet and Alzheimer disease mortality." Neurology. 69: 1084–1093 (2007)

Scarmeas N, Luchsinger JA, Stern Y, Gu Y, He J, DeCarli C, Brown T, and Brickman AM. "Mediterranean diet and magnetic resonance imaging-assessed cerebrovascular disease." Ann Neurol 69: 257–268 (2011)

Serra-Majem L, Roman B, and Estruch R. "Scientific evidence of interventions using the Mediterranean diet: a systematic review." Nutr Rev 64: S27–S47 (2006)

Shai I, Schwarzfuchs D, Henkin Y, Shahar DR, Witkow S, Greenberg I, Golan R, Fraser D, Bolotin A, Vardi H, Tangi-Rozental O, Zuk-Ramot R, Sarusi B, Brickner D, Schwartz Z, Sheiner E, Marko R, Katorza E, Thiery J, Fiedler GM, Blüher M, Stumvoll M, and Stampfer MJ. "Dietary Intervention Randomized Controlled Trial (DIRECT) Group. "Weight loss with a low-carbohydrate, Mediterranean, or low-fat diet." N Engl J Med 359: 229–241 (2008)

Siri-Tarino PW, Sun Q, Hu FB, and Krauss RM. "Meta-analysis of prospective cohort studies evaluating the association of saturated fat with cardiovascular disease." Am J Clin Nutr 91: 535–546 (2010)

Singh B, Parsaik AK, Mielke MM, Erwin PJ, Knopman DS, Petersen RC and Roberts RO. "Association of Mediterranean diet with mild cognitive impairment and Alzheimer's disease." J Alzheimer's Dis 39: 271–282 (2013)

Sjogren P, Becker W, Warensjö E, Olsson E, Byberg L, Gustafsson IB, Karlström B, and Cederholm T. "Mediterranean and carbohydrate-restricted diets and mortality among elderly men: a cohort study in Sweden." Am J Clin Nutr 92: 967–974 (2010)

Sofi F, Macchi C, Abbate R, Gensini GF, and Casini A. "Effectiveness of the Mediterranean diet: can it help delay or prevent Alzheimer's disease?" J Alzheimer's Dis 20: 795–801 (2010)

Tangney CC, Kwasny MJ, Li H, Wilson RS, Evans DA, and Morris MC. "Adherence to a Mediterranean-type dietary pattern and cognitive decline in a community population." Am J Clin Nutr 93: 601–607 (2011)

Tognon G, Kwasny MJ, Li H, Wilson RS, Evans DA, and Morris MC. "Does the Mediterranean diet predict longevity in the elderly? A Swedish perspective." Age 33: 439–450 (2011)

Trichopoulou A, Costacou T, Bamia C, and Trichopoulos D. "Adherence to a Mediterranean diet and survival in a Greek population." N Engl J Med 348: 2599–2608 (2003)

Trichopoulo A, Naska A, Orfanos P, and Trichopoulos D. "Mediterranean diet in relation to body mass index and waist-to-hip ratio: the Greek European Prospective Investigation into Cancer and Nutrition Study." Am J Clin Nutr 82: 935–40 (2005)

Tsivgoulis G, Judd S, Letter AJ, Alexandrov AV, Howard G, Nahab F, Unverzagt FW, Moy C, Howard VJ, Kissela B, and Wadley VG. "Adherence to a Mediterranean diet and risk of incident cognitive impairment." Neurology 80: 1684–1692 (2013)

Valls-Pedret C, Lamuela-Raventós RM, Medina-Remón A, Quintana M, Corella D, Pintó X, Martínez-González MÁ, Estruch R, and Ros E. "Polyphenol-rich foods in the Mediterranean diet are associated with better cognitive function in elderly subjects at high cardiovascular risk." J Alzheimer's Dis 29: 773–782 (2012)

Vassallo N and Scerri C. "Mediterranean diet and dementia of the Alzheimer type." Curr Aging Sci 6: 150–162 (2013)

Vasto S, Scapagnini G, Rizzo C, Monastero R, Marchese A, and Caruso C. "Mediterranean diet and longevity in Sicily: survey in a Sicani Mountains population." Rejuvenation Res 15: 184–188 (2012)

Willett WC, Sacks F, Trichopoulou A, Drescher G, Ferro-Luzzi A, Helsing E, and Trichopoulos D. "Mediterranean diet pyramid: a cultural model for healthy eating." Am J Clin Nutr 61: 1402–1406S (1995)

CHAPTER 6. ANTI-INFLAMMATORY SUPPLEMENTS

Chung S, Yao H, Caito S, Hwang JW, Arunachalam G, and Rahman I. "Regulation of SIRT1 in cellular functions: role of polyphenols." Arch Biochem Biophys 501: 79–90 (2010)

Consumer Reports. "Fish oil pills vs. claims." January, 2012 (2012)

Depner CM, Taber MG, bobe G, Kensicki E, Bohren KM, and Jump DB. "A metabolomics analysis of omega-3 fatty acid-mediated attenuation of Western diet-induced nonalcoholic steatohaptitis in LDLR-/- mice." PLoS ONE 8: e83756 (2013)

Easton MDL, Luszniak D, and E Von der Geest. "Preliminary examination of contaminant loadings in farmed salmon, wild salmon and commercial salmon feed." Chemosphere 46: 1053–1074 (2002)

Endres S, Ghorbani R, Kelley VE, Georgilis K, Lonnemann G, van der Meer JW, Cannon JG, Rogers TS, Klempner MS, Weber PC, Schafter EJ, Wolff SM, and Dinarello CA. "The effect of dietary supplementation with n-3 polyunsaturated fatty acids on the synthesis of interleukin-1 and tumor necrosis factor by mononuclear cells." N Engl J Med 320: 265–271 (1989)

Freeman D. "American Kids Aren't the Fattest After All: Go Spain and Italy!" CBS News (http: //www.cbsnews.com/news/american-kids-arent-the-fattest-after-all-go-spain-and-italy). June 25, 2010 (2010)

Haorah J, Knipe B, Leibhart J, Ghorpade A, and Persidsky Y. "Alcohol-induced oxidative stress in brain endothelial cells causes blood-brain barrier dysfunction." J Leukoc Biol 78: 1223–1232 (2005)

Harris WS, Pottala JV, Varvel SA, Borowski JJ, Ward JN, and McConnell JP. "Erythrocyte omega-3 fatty acids increase and linoleic acid decreases with age: observations from 160,000 patients." Prostaglandins Leukot Essent Fatty Acids 88: 257–263 (2013)

Holub DJ and Holub BJ. "Omega-3 fatty acids from fish oils and cardiovascular disease." Mol Cell Biochem 263: 217–225 (2004)

Hwang JT, Kwon DY, and Yoon SH. "AMP-activated protein kinase: a potential target for the diseases prevention by natural occurring polyphenols." N Biotechnol 26: 17–22 (2009)

Kawabata T, Hirota S, Hirayama T, Adachi N, Hagiwara C, Iwama N, Kamachi K, Araki E, Kawashima H, and Kiso Y. "Age-related changes of dietary intake and blood eicosapentaenoic acid, docosahexaenoic acid, and arachidonic acid levels in Japanese men and women." Prostaglandins Leukot Essent Fatty Acids 84: 131–137 (2011)

Kiecolt-Glaser JK, Epel ES, Belury MA, Andridge R, Lin J, Glaser R, Malarkey WB, Hwang BS, and Blackburn E. "Omega-3 fatty acids, oxidative stress, and leukocyte telomere length: A randomized controlled trial." Brain Behav Immun 28: 16–24 (2013)

MacFarlane N, Salt J, Birkin R and Kendrick A. "The FAST Index - a fishy scale. A search for a test to quantify fish flavor." INFORM 12: 244–249 (2001)

Mueller T. *Extra Virginity: The Sublime and Scandalous World of Olive Oil.* W.W. Norton. New York, NY (2011)

Perez-Jimenez J, Neveu V, Vos F, and Scalbert A. "Identification of the 100 richest dietary sources of polyphenols." Eur J Clin Nutr 64: S112–S120 (2010)

Rizzo AM, Montorfano G, Negroni M, Adorni L, Berselli P, Corsetto P, Wahle K, and Berra B. "A rapid method for determining arachidonic: eicosapentaenoic acid ratios in whole blood lipids: correlation with erythrocyte membrane ratios and validation in a large Italian population of various ages and pathologies." Lipids Health Dis 9: 7 (2010)

Sears, B. *The OmegaRx Zone.* Regan Books. New York, NY (2002)

CHAPTER 7: POLYPHENOLS: THE NEXT ESSENTIAL NUTRIENTS

Andujar I, Recio MC, Giner RM, and Rios JL. "Cocoa polyphenols and their potential benefits for human health." Oxid Med Cell Longev 2012: 906252 (2012)

Christaki E and Opal SM. "Is the mortality rate for septic shock really decreasing?" Curr Opin Crit Care 14: 580–586 (2008)

Daglia M. "Polyphenols as antimicrobial agents." Curr Opin Biotechnol 23: 174–181 (2012)

Faller ALK and Fialho E. "Polyphenol content and antioxidant capacity in organic and conventional plant foods." J Food Composition and Analysis 23: 561–568 (2010)

Frankenburg FR. *Vitamin Discoveries and Disasters: History, Science, and Controversies.* Praeger Press. Westport, CT. (2009)

Hwang JT, Kwon DY, and Yoon SH. "AMP-activated protein kinase: a potential target for the diseases prevention by natural occurring polyphenols." N Biotechnol 26: 17–22 (2009)

Lippi D. "Chocolate in history: food, medicine, medi-food." Nutrients 5: 1573–1585 (2013)

Landete JM. "Updated knowledge about polyphenols: functions, bioavailability, metabolism, and health." Crit Rev Food Sci Nutr 52: 936–948 (2012)

Miller KB, Hurst WJ, Flannigan N, Ou B, Lee CY, Smith N, and Stuart DA. "Survey of commercially available chocolate- and cocoa-containing products in the United States. Comparison of flavan-3-ol content with nonfat cocoa solids, total polyphenols, and percent cacao." J Agric Food Chem 57: 9169–9180 (2009)

Obrenovich ME, Nair NG, Beyaz A, Aliev G, and Reddy VP. "The role of polyphenolic antioxidants in health, disease, and aging." Rejuvenation Res 13: 631–643 (2010)

Perez-Jimenez J, Neveu V, Vos F, and Scalbert A. "Identification of the 100 richest dietary sources of polyphenols." Eur J Clin Nutr 64: S112–S120 (2010)

Rawel HW and Kulling SE. "Nutritional contribution of coffee, cocoa, and tea phenolics to human health." J Consumer Protection and Food Safety 2: 399–407 (2007)

Scapagnini G, Vasto S, Abraham NG, Caruso C, Zella D, and Fabio G. "Modulation of Nrf2/ARE pathway by food polyphenols: a nutritional neuroprotective strategy for cognitive and neurodegenerative disorders." Mol Neurobiol 44: 192–201 (2011)

Scholz S and Williamson G. "Interactions affecting the bioavailability of dietary polyphenols in vivo." Int J Vitam Nutr Res 77: 224–235 (2007)

Visioli F, De La Lastra CA, Andres-Lacueva C, Aviram M, Calhau C, Cassano A, D'Archivio M, Faria A, Fave G, Fogliano V, Llorach R, Vitaglione P, Zoratti M, and Edeas M. "Polyphenols and human health: a prospectus." Crit Rev Food Sci Nutr 51: 524–546 (2011)

Wilson PK and Hurst WJ. *Chocolate as Medicine.* RSC Publishers. Cambridge, UK (2012)

CHAPTER 8: POLYPHENOLS AND GUT HEALTH

Cardona F, Andres-Lacueva C, Tulipani S, Tinahones FJ, and Queipo-Ortuno MI. "Benefits of polyphenols on gut microbiota and implications in human health." J Nutr Biochem 24: 1415–1422 (2013)

Caricilli AM and Saad MJ. "The role of gut microbiota on insulin resistance." Nutrients 5: 829–851 (2013)

Clemente JC, Ursell LK, Parfrey LW, and Knight R. "The impact of the gut microbiota on human health: an integrative view." Cell 148: 1258–1270 (2012)

Davis JE, Gabler NK, Walker-Daniels J, and Spurlock ME. "TLR-4 deficiency selectively protects against obesity induced by diets high in saturated fat." Obesity 16: 1248–1255 (2008)

Fresno M, Alvarez R, and Cuesta N. "Toll-like receptors, inflammation, metabolism and obesity." Arch Physiol Biochem 117: 151–164 (2011)

Gershon M. *The Second Brain*. Harper Perennial. New York, NY (1999)

Kayama H and Takeda K. "Regulation of intestinal homeostasis by innate and adaptive immunity." Int Immunol 24: 673–680 (2012)

Kennedy P. "The Fat Drug." New York Times. March 8, 2014 (2014)

Kim JJ and Sears DD. "TLR4 and insulin resistance." Gastroenterol Res Pract 2010: S1687 (2010)

David LA, Maurice CF, Carmody RN, Gootenberg DB, Button JE, Wolfe BE, Ling AV, Devlin AS, Varma Y, Fischbach MA, Biddinger SB, Dutton RJ, and Turnbaugh PJ. "Diet rapidly and reproducibly alters the human gut microbiome." Nature 505: 559–563 (2014)

Ley RE, Turnbaugh PJ, Klein S, and Gordon JI. "Microbial ecology: human gut microbes associated with obesity." Nature 444: 1022–1023 (2006)

Mirsky, S. "2011 Nobel Prize in Physiology or Medicine." Scientific American October 3, 2011 (2011)

Rodriguez-Lagunas MJ, Storniolo CE, Ferrer R, and Moreno JJ. "5-hydroxyeicosatetraenoic acid and leukotriene D4 increase intestinal epithelial paracellular permeability." Int J Biochem Cell Biol 45: 1318–1326 (2013)

Shi H, Kokoeva MV, Inouye K, Tzameli I, Yin H, and Flier JS. "TLR4 links innate immunity and fatty acid-induced insulin resistance." J Clin Invest 116: 3015–3025 (2006)

Sykes B. *The Seven Daughters of Eve*. W. W. Norton. New York, NY (2002)

van Houte J and Gibbons RJ. "Studies of the cultivable flora of normal human feces." Antonie van Leeuwenhoek 32: 212–222 (1966)

Watanabe Y, Nagai Y, and Takatsu K. "Activation and regulation of the pattern recognition receptors in obesity-induced adipose tissue inflammation and insulin resistance." Nutrients 5: 3757–3778 (2013)

Zhang X, Zhang G, Zhang H, Karin M, Bai H, and Cai D. "Hypothalamic IKKbeta/NF-kappaB and ER stress link overnutrition to energy imbalance and obesity." Cell 135: 61–73 (2008)

CHAPTER 9: POLYPHENOLS AND OXIDATIVE STRESS

Basu A, Du M, Leyva MJ, Sanchez K, Betts NM, Wu M, Aston CE, and Lyons TJ. "Blueberries decrease cardiovascular risk factors in obese men and women with metabolic syndrome." J Nutr 140: 1582–1587 (2010)

Cao G, Booth SL, Sadowski JA, and Prior RL. "Increases in human plasma antioxidant capacity after consumption of controlled diets high in fruit and vegetables." Am J Clin Nutr 68: 1081–1087 (1998)

Chen CY, Yi L, Jin X, Mi MT, Zhang T, Ling WH, and Yu B. "Delphinidin attenuates stress injury induced by oxidized low-density lipoprotein in human umbilical vein endothelial cells." Chem Biol Interact 183: 105–112 (2010)

Conklin KA. "Dietary antioxidants during cancer chemotherapy: impact on chemotherapeutic effectiveness and development of side effects." Nutrition and Cancer 37: 1–18 (2000)

Erlank H, Elmann A, Kohen R, and Kanner J. "Polyphenols activate Nrf2 in astrocytes via H2O2, semiquinones, and quinones." Free Radic Biol Med 51: 2319–27 (2011)

Holvoet P. "Oxidized LDL and coronary heart disease." Acta Cardiol 59: 479–484 (2004)

Hybertson BM, Gao B, Bose SK, and McCord JM. "Oxidative stress in health and disease: the therapeutic potential of Nrf2 activation." Mol Aspects Med 32: 234–246 (2011)

Krikorian R, Shidler MD, Nash TA, Kalt W, Vinqvist-Tymchuk MR, Shukitt-Hale B, and Joseph JA. "Blueberry supplementation improves memory in older adults." J Agric Food Chem 58: 3996–4000 (2010)

Knight JA. "Review: Free radicals, antioxidants, and the immune system." Ann Clin Lab Sci 30: 145–158 (2000)

Li Y, Daniel M, and Tollefsbol TO. "Epigenetic regulation of caloric restriction in aging." BMC Med 9: 98 (2011)

Li W, Khor TO, Xu C, Shen G, Jeong WS, Yu S, and Kong AN. "Activation of Nrf2-antioxidant signaling attenuates NF-kappaB-inflammatory response and elicits apoptosis." Biochem Pharmacol 76: 1485–1489 (2008)

Manach C, Scalbert A, Morand C, Remesy C, and Jimenez L. "Polyphenols: food sources and bioavailability." Am J Clin Nutr 79: 727–747 (2004)

Nathan C. "Points of control in inflammation." Nature 420: 846–852 (2002)

Nathan C and Ding A. "Nonresolving inflammation." Cell 140: 871–882 (2010)

Prior RL, Cao G, Prior RL, and Cao G. "Analysis of botanicals and dietary supplements for antioxidant capacity: a review." J AOAC Int 83: 950–956 (2000)

Scapagnini G, Vasto S, Abraham NG, Caruso C, Zella D, and Fabio G. "Modulation of Nrf2/ARE pathway by food polyphenols: a nutritional neuroprotective strategy for cognitive and neurodegenerative disorders." Mol Neurobiol 44: 192–201 (2011)

Scholz S and Williamson G. "Interactions affecting the bioavailability of dietary polyphenols in vivo." Int J Vitam Nutr Res 77: 224–235 (2007)

Sears B. The Anti-Aging Zone. Regan Books. New York, NY (1999)

Spite M, Claria J, and Serhan CN. "Resolvins, specialized proresolving lipid mediators and their potential roles in metabolic diseases." Cell Metabolism 19: 21–36 (2014)

Wallace SS. "Biological consequences of free radical-damaged DNA bases." Free Radic Biol Med 33: 1–14 (2002)

Zhang MJ and Spite M. "Resolvins: anti-inflammatory and proresolving mediators derived from omega-3 polyunsaturated fatty acids." Annu Rev Nutr 32: 203–227 (2012)

U.S. FDA. "FDA expands advice on statin risk." www.fda.gov/forconsumers/consumerupdates/ucm293330.htm#2

CHAPTER 10: POLYPHENOLS AND LONGEVITY

Anderson RM and Weindruch R. "Metabolic reprogramming, caloric restriction and aging." Trends Endocrinol Metab 21: 134–141 (2010)

Ayissi VB, Ebrahimi A, and Schluesenner H. "Epigenetic effects of natural polyphenols: A focus on SIRT1-mediated mechanisms." Mol Nutr Food Res 58: 22–32 (2014)

Bao Y, Han J, Hu FB, Giovannucci EL, Stampfer MJ, Willett WC, and Fuchs SC. "Association of nut consumption with total and cause-specific mortality." N Engl J Med 369: 2001–2011 (2013)

Cassidy A, Mukamal KJ, Liu L, Franz M, Eliassen AH and EB. "High anthocyanin intake is associated with a reduced risk of myocardial infarction in young and middle-aged women." Circulation 127: 188–196 (2013)

Chang HC and Guarente L. "SIRT1 and other sirtuins in metabolism." Trends Endocrinol Metab 25: 138–145 (2014)

Chung S, Yao H, Caito S, Hwang JW, Arunachalam G, and Rahman I. "Regulation of SIRT1 in cellular functions: role of polyphenols." Arch Biochem Biophys 501: 79–90 (2010)

Fontana L. "The scientific basis of caloric restriction leading to longer life." Curr Opin Gastroenterol 25: 144–150 (2009)

Goldman DP, Cutler D, Rowe JW, Michaud P, Sullivan, J, Peneva K, and Olshansky SJ. "Substantial health and economic returns from delayed aging may warrant a new focus for medical research." Health Affairs 32: 1698–1705 (2013)

Holloszy JO and Fontana L. "Caloric restriction in humans." Exp Gerontol 42: 709–712 (2007)

Hou X, Xu S, Maitland-Toolan KA, Sato K, Jiang B, Ido Y, Lan F, Walsh K, Wierzbicki M, Verbeuren TJ, Cohen RA, and Zang M. "SIRT1 regulates hepatocyte lipid metabolism through activating AMP-activated protein kinase." J Biol Chem 283: 20015–20026 (2008)

Hwang JT, Kwon DY, and Yoon SH. "AMP-activated protein kinase: a potential target for the diseases prevention by natural occurring polyphenols." Nature Biotechnol 26: 17–22 (2009)

McCay CM, Crowell MF, Maynard LA. "The effect of retarded growth upon the length of life span and upon the ultimate body size." J Nutr 10: 63–79 (1935)

Sears B. The Anti-Aging Zone. Regan Books. New York, NY (1999)

Tennen RI, Michishita-Kioi E,and Chua KF. "Finding a target for resveratrol." Cell 148: 387–389 (2012)

Tollefsbol T (ed). Epigenetics in Human Disease. Academic Press. New York, NY (2012)

Zamora-Ros R, Rabassa M, Cherubini A, Urpí-Sardà M, Bandinelli S, Ferrucci L, Andres-Lacueva C. "High concentrations of a urinary biomarker of polyphenol intake are associated with decreased mortality in older adults." J Nutr 143: 1445–1450 (2013)

CHAPTER 11: THE INDUSTRIALIZATION OF FOOD AND THE RISE OF INFLAMMATION

Avena NM, Rada P, and Hoebel BG. "Evidence for sugar addiction: behavioral and neurochemical effects of intermittent, excessive sugar intake." Neurosci Biobehav Rev 32: 20–39 (2008)

Bachmanov AA and Beauchamp GK. "Taste receptor genes." Annu Rev Nutr 27: 389–414 (2007)

Breslin PA and Beauchamp GK. "Salt enhances flavour by suppressing bitterness." Nature 387: 563 (1997)

Irie F, Fitzpatrick AL, Lopez OL, Kuller LH, Peila R, Newman AB, and Launer LJ. "Enhanced risk for Alzheimer disease in persons with type 2 diabetes and APOE epsilon4: the Cardiovascular Health Study Cognition Study." Arch Neurol 65: 89–93 (2008)

Lenoir M, Serre F, Cantin L, and Ahmed SH. "Intense sweetness surpasses cocaine reward." PLoS ONE 2: e698 (2007)

Mehla J, Chauhan BC, and Chauhan NB. "Experimental induction of type 2 diabetes in aging-accelerated mice triggered Alzheimer-like pathology and memory deficits." J Alzheimer's Dis 39: 145–162 (2014)

Moss M. *Salt Sugar Fat: How the Food Giants Hooked Us.* Random House, NY (2013)

Mozaffarian D, Pischon T, Hankinson SE, Rifai N, Joshipura K, Willett WC, and Rimm EB. "Dietary intake of trans fatty acids and systemic inflammation in women." Am J Clin Nutr 79: 606–612 (2004)

Mozaffarian D, Aro A, and Willett WC. "Health effects of trans-fatty acids: experimental and observational evidence." Eur J Clin Nutr 63: S5–21 (2009)

Profenno LA, Porsteinsson AP, and Faraone SV. "Meta-analysis of Alzheimer's disease risk with obesity, diabetes, and related disorders." Biol Psychiatry 67: 505–512 (2010)

Siri-Tarino PW, Sun Q; Hu FB, and Krauss RM. "Meta-analysis of prospective cohort studies evaluating the association of saturated fat with cardiovascular disease." Am J Clin Nutr 91: 535–546 (2010)

Spangler R, Wittkowski KM, Goddard NL, Avena NM, Hoebel BG, and Leibowitz SF. "Opiate-like effects of sugar on gene expression in reward areas of the rat brain." Brain Res Mol Brain Res 124: 134–142 (2004)

Spetter MS, Smeets PA, de Graaf C, and Viergever MA. "Representation of sweet and salty taste intensity in the brain." Chem Senses 35: 831–840 (2010)

Xu Y, Wang L, He J, Bi Y, Li M, Wang T, Wang L, Jiang Y. Dai M, Lu J, Xu M, Li Y, Hu N, Li J, Mi S, Chen CS, Li G, Mu Y, Zhao J, Kong L, Chen J, Lai S, Wang W, Zhao W, and Ning G. "Prevalence and control of diabetes in Chinese adults." JAMA 310: 948–959 (2013)

Zhu X, Tang X, Anderson VE, and Sayre LM. "Mass spectrometric characterization of protein modification by the products of nonenzymatic oxidation of linoleic acid." Chem Res Toxicol 22: 1386–1397 (2009)

CHAPTER 12: CHASING THE WRONG FOOD VILLAINS

American Heart Association. "Dietary guidelines for healthy American adults." Circulation 77: 721A–724A (1988)

Berg JM, Tymoczko JL, and Stryer L. *Biochemistry, 5th edition.* W.H. Freeman. New York, NY (2002)

Beguin P, Errachid A, Larondelle Y, and Schneider YJ. "Effect of polyunsaturated fatty acids on tight junctions in a model of the human intestinal epithelium under normal and inflammatory conditions." Food Funct 4: 923–931 (2013)

Brouns F, van Buul VJ, and Shewry PR. "Does wheat make us fat and sick?" J Cereal Sci 58: 209–213 (2013)

Bray GA, Nielsen SJ, and Popkin BM. "Consumption of high-fructose corn syrup in beverages may play a role in the epidemic of obesity." Am J Clin Nutr 79: 537–543 (2004)

Butterwoth T. "Sweet and Sour: The media decided fructose was bad for America, but science had second thoughts." Forbes February 6, 2014 (2014)

Carden TJ and Carr TP. "Food availability of glucose and fat, but not fructose, increased in the US between 1970 and 2009." Nutr J 12: 130 (2013)

Cavalli-Sforza LT, Strata A, Barone A, and Cucurachi L. "Primary adult lactose malabsorption in Italy: regional differences in prevalence and relationship to lactose intolerance and milk consumption." Am J Clin Nutr 45: 748–754 (1987)

Cook HW. "The influence of trans-acids on desaturation and elongation of fatty acids in developing brain." Lipids 16: 920–926 (1981)

Cook HW and Emken EA. "Geometric and positional fatty acid isomers interact differently with desaturation and elongation of linoleic and linolenic acids in cultured glioma cells." Biochem Cell Biol 68: 653–660 (1990)

Crittenden RG and Bennett LE. "Cow's milk allergy: A complex disorder." Journal of the American College of Nutrition 24: 582S–591S (2005)

Cruz-Teno C, Perez-Martinez P, Delgado-Lista J, Yubero-Serrano EM, Garcia-Rios A, Marin C, Gomez P, Jimenez-Gomez Y, Camargo A, Rodriguez-Cantalejo F, Malagon MM, Perez-Jimenez F, Roche HM, and Lopez-Miranda J. "Dietary fat modifies the postprandial inflammatory state in subjects with metabolic syndrome: the LIPGENE study." Mol Nutr Food Res 56: 854–865 (2012)

Davis JE, Gabler NK, Walker-Daniels J, and Spurlock ME. "TLR-4 deficiency selectively protects against obesity induced by diets high in saturated fat." Obesity 16: 1248–1255 (2008)

Davis W. *Wheat Belly: Lose the Wheat, Lose the Weight, and Find Your Path Back to Health.* Rodale Books. Erasmus, PA (2011)

de Lorgeril M, Renaud S, Mamelle N, Salen P, Martin JL, Monjaud I, Guidollet J, Touboul P, and Delaye J. "Mediterranean alpha-linolenic acid-rich diet in secondary prevention of coronary heart disease." Lancet 343: 1454–1459 (1994)

de Lorgeril M. Salen P, Martin JL, Monjaud I, Delaye J, and Mamelle N. "Mediterranean diet, traditional risk factors, and the rate of cardiovascular complications after myocardial infarction: final report of the Lyon Diet Heart Study." Circulation 99: 779–785 (1999)

Ghosh S, Mocan E, DeCoffe D, Dai C, and Gibson D. "Diets rich in n-6 PUFA induce intestinal microbioal dysbiosis in aged mice." Brit J Nutr 110: 515–523 (2013)

Fasano A. *Gluten Freedom: The Nation's Leading Expert Offers the Essential Guide to a Healthy, Gluten-Free Lifestyle.* Wiley. New York, NY (2014)

Ebbeling CB, Swain JF, Feldman HA, Wong WW, Hachey DL, Garcia-Lago E, and Ludwig DS. "Effects of dietary composition on energy expenditure during weight-loss maintenance." JAMA 307: 2627–2634 (2012)

Enos RT, Davis JM, Velazquez KT, McClellan JL, Day SD, Carnevale KA, and Murphy EA. "Influence of dietary saturated fat content on adiposity, macrophage behavior, inflammation, and metabolism: composition matters." J Lipid Res 54: 152–163 (2013)

Kennedy A, Martinez K, Chuang C, LaPost K, and McIntosh M. "Saturated fatty acid-mediated inflammation and insulin resistance in the adipose tissue." J Nutr 139: 1–4 (2009)

Kien CL, Bunn JY, Tompkins CL, Dumas JA, Crain KI, Ebenstein DB, Koves TR, and Muoio DM. "Substituting dietary monounsaturated fat for saturated fat is associated with increased daily physical activity and resting energy expenditure and with changes in mood." Am J Clin Nutr 97: 689–697 (2013)

Kuipers RS, de Graaf DJ, Luxwolda MF, Muskiet MH, Dijck-Brouwer DA, and Muskiet FA. "Saturated fat, carbohydrates and cardiovascular disease." Neth J Med 69: 372–378 (2011)

Klurfeld DM, Foreyt J, Angelopoulos TJ, and Rippe JM. "Lack of evidence for high fructose corn syrup as the cause of the obesity epidemic." Int J Obes 37: 771–773 (2013)

Harris WS, Mozaffarian D, Rimm E, Kris-Etherton P, Rudel LL, Appel LJ, Engler MM, Engler MB, and Sacks F. "Omega-6 fatty acids and risk for cardiovascular disease: a science advisory from the American Heart Association Nutrition Subcommittee of the Council on Nutrition, Physical Activity, and Metabolism; Council on Cardiovascular Nursing; and Council on Epidemiology and Prevention." Circulation 119: 902–907 (2009)

Hill EG, Johnson SB, Lawson LD, Mahfouz MM, and Holman RT. "Perturbation of the metabolism of essential fatty acids by dietary partially hydrogenated vegetable oil." Proc Natl Acad Sci USA 79: 953–957 (1982)

Holt SHA, Brand-Miller JC, and Petocz. "An insulin index of foods." Am J Clin Nutr 66: 1264–1276 (1997)

Hoyt G, Hickey MS, and Cordain L. "Dissociation of the glycaemic and insulinaemic responses to whole and skimmed milk." Br J Nutr 93: 175–177 (2005)

Host A. "Frequency of cow's milk allergy in childhood." Ann Allergy Asthma Immunol 89: 33–37 (2002)

Hokayem M, Blond E, Vidal H, Lambert K, Meugnier E, Feillet-Coudray C, Coudray C, Pesenti S, Luyton C, Lambert-Porcheron S, Sauvinet V, Fedou C, Brun JF, Rieusset J, Bisbal C, Sultan A, Mercier J, Goudable J, Dupuy AM, Cristol JP, Laville M, and Avignon A. "Grape polyphenols prevent fructose-induced oxidative stress and insulin resistance in first-degree relatives of type 2 diabetic patients." Diabetes Care 2013 36: 1454–1461 (2013)

Jayashree B, Bibin YS, Prabhu D, Shanthirani CS, Gokulakrishnan K, Lakshmi BS, Mohan V, and Balasubramanyam M. "Increased circulatory levels of lipopolysaccharide (LPS) and zonulin signify novel biomarkers of proinflammation in patients with type 2 diabetes." Mol Cell Biochem 388: 203–210 (2014)

Johnston CS, Tjonn SL, Swan PD, White A, Hutchins H, and Sears B. "Ketogenic low-carbohydrate diets have no metabolic advantage over nonketogenic low-carbohydrate diets." Am J Clin Nutr 83: 1055–1061 (2006)

Liebman B. "The changing American diet." Nutritional Action Newsletter. September, 2013 (http://cspinet.org/new/pdf/changing_american_diet_13.pdf) (2013)

Lopez-Garcia E, Schulze MB, Meigs JB, Manson JE, Rifai N, Stampfer MJ, Willett WC, and Hu FB. "Consumption of trans fatty acids is related to plasma biomarkers of inflammation and endothelial dysfunction." J Nutr 135: 562–566 (2005)

Lopez S, Bermudez B, Ortega A, Varela LM, Pacheco YM, Villar J, Abia R, and Muriana FJ. "Effects of meals rich in either monounsaturated or saturated fat on lipid concentrations and on insulin secretion and action in subjects with high fasting triglyceride concentrations." Am J Clin Nutr 93: 494–499 (2011)

Lowndes J, Kawiecki D, Pardo S, Nguyen V, Melanson KJ, Yu Z, and Rippe JM. "The effects of four hypocaloric diets containing different levels of sucrose or high fructose corn syrup on weight loss and related parameters." Nutr J 11: 55 (2012)

Lustig RH. *Fat Chance: Beating the Odds Against Sugar, Processed Food, Obesity, and Disease.* Hudson Street Press. New York, NY (2012)

Maric T, Woodside B, and Luhenshi GN. "The effects of dietary saturated fat on basal hypothalamic neuroinflammation in rats." Brain Behave Immun 36: 35–45 (2014)

Massoumi R and Sjolander A. "The inflammatory mediator leukotriene D4 triggers a rapid reorganisation of the actin cytoskeleton in human intestinal epithelial cells." Eur J Cell Biol 76: 185–191 (1998)

Mensink RP and Katan MB. "Effect of dietary trans fatty acids on high-density and low-density lipoprotein cholesterol levels in healthy subjects." N Engl J Med 323: 439–445 (1990)

Moss M. *Salt Sugar Fat: How the Food Giants Hooked Us.* Random House, NY (2013)

Mozaffarian D, Aro A, and Willett WC. "Health effects of trans-fatty acids: experimental and observational evidence." Eur J Clin Nutr 63: S5–S21 (2009)

Perlmutter D. *Grain Brain: The Surprising Truth about Wheat, Carbs, and Sugar-Your Brain's Silent Killers.* Little, Brown and Company. New York, NY (2013)

Poledne R. "A new atherogenetic effect of saturated fatty acids." Physiol Res 62: 139–143 (2013)

Ramsden CE, Hibbeln JR, Majchrzak SF, and Davis JM. "n-6 fatty acid-specific and mixed polyunsaturate dietary interventions have different effects on CHD risk: a meta-analysis of randomised controlled trials." Br J Nutr 104: 1586–600 (2010)

Ramsden CE, Zamora D, Leelarthaepin B, Majchrzak-Hong SF, Faurot KR, Suchindran CM, Ringel A, Davis JM, and Hibbeln JR. "Use of dietary linoleic acid for secondary prevention of coronary heart disease and death: evaluation of recovered data from the Sydney Diet Heart Study and updated meta-analysis." BMJ 346: e8707 (2013)

Ratnesar R. "Against the Grain." Time. December 15, 1997 (1997)

Raz O, Steinvil A, Berliner S, Rosenzweig T, Justo D, and Shapira I. "The effect of two iso-caloric meals containing equal amounts of fats with a different fat composition on the inflammatory and metabolic markers in apparently healthy volunteers." J Inflamm 10: 3 (2013)

Rippe JM and Angelopoulos TJ. "Sucrose, high-fructose corn syrup, and fructose their metabolism and potential health effects: What do we really know?" Adv Nutr 4: 236–245 (2013)

Roach C, Feller SE, Ward JA, Shaikh SR, Zerouga M, and Stillwell W. "Comparison of cis and trans fatty acid containing phosphatidylcholines on membrane properties." Biochemistry 43: 6344–6351 (2004)

Sievenpiper JL, de Souza RJ, Mirrahimi A, Yu ME, Carleton AJ, Beyene J, Chiavaroli L, Di Buono M, Jenkins AL, Leiter LA, Wolever TM, Kendall CW, and Jenkins DJ. "Effect of fructose on body weight in controlled feeding trials: a systematic review and meta-analysis." Ann Intern Med 156: 291–304 (2012)

Sievenpiper JL, Chiavaroli L, de Souza RJ, Mirrahimi A, Cozma AI, Ha V, Wang DD, Yu ME, Carleton AJ, Beyene J, Di Buono M, Jenkins AL, Leiter LA, Wolever TM, Kendall CW, and Jenkins DJ. "Catalytic doses of fructose may benefit glycaemic control without harming cardiometabolic risk factors: a small meta-analysis of randomised controlled feeding trials." Br J Nutr 108: 418–423 (2012)

Sievenpiper JL, de Souza RJ, Cozma AI, Chavaroli L, Ha V, and Mirrhimi A. "Fructose vs. glucose and metabolism." Current Opin Lipidology 25: 8–19 (2014)

Silk DB, Grimble GK, and Rees RG. "Protein digestion and amino acid and peptide absorption." Proc Nutr Soc 44: 63–72 (1985)

Siri-Tarino PW, Sun Q, Hu FB, and Krauss RM. "Meta-analysis of prospective cohort studies evaluating the association of saturated fat with cardiovascular disease." Am J Clin Nutr 91: 535–546 (2010)

Sundram K, Karupaiah T, and Hayes KC. "Stearic acid-rich interesterified fat and trans-rich fat raise the LDL/HDL ratio and plasma glucose relative to palm olein in humans." Nutr Metab 4: 3 (2007)

Wang D, Sievenpiper JL, de Souza RJ, Cozma AI, Chiavaroli L, Ha V, Mirrahimi A, Carleton AJ, Di Buono M, Jenkins AL, Leiter LA, Wolever TM, Beyene J, Kendall CW, and Jenkins D. "Effect of fructose on postprandial triglycerides: A systematic review and meta-analysis of controlled feeding trials." Atherosclerosis 232: 125–133 (2014)

White JS. "Challenging the fructose hypothesis." Adv Nutr 4: 246–256 (2013)

CHAPTER 13: EPIGENETICS: OPENING PANDORA'S GENETIC BOX

Ailhaud G, Massiera F, Weill P, Legrand P, Alessandri JM, and Guesnet P. "Temporal changes in dietary fats: role of n-6 polyunsaturated fatty acids in excessive adipose tissue development and relationship to obesity." Prog Lipid Res 45: 203–206 (2006)

Ailhaud G, Guesnet P, and Cunnane SC. "An emerging risk factor for obesity: does disequilibrium of polyunsaturated fatty acid metabolism contribute to excessive adipose tissue development?" Br J Nutr 100: 461–470 (2008)

Ailhaud G. "Omega-6 fatty acids and excessive adipose tissue development." World Rev Nutr Diet 98: 51–61 (2008)

Alvheim AR, Malde MK, Osei-Hyiaman D, Lin YH, Pawlosky RJ, Madsen L, Kristiansen K, Froyland L, and Hibbeln JR. "Dietary linoleic acid elevates endogenous 2-AG and anandamide and induces obesity." Obesity 10: 1984–1994 (2012)

Alvheim AR, Torstensen BE, Lin YH, Lillefosse HH, Lock EJ, Madsen L, Froyland L,

Hibbeln JR, and Malde MK. "Dietary linoleic acid elevates the endocannabinoids 2-AG and anandamide and promotes weight gain in mice fed a low fat diet." Lipids 49: 59–69 (2014)

Bayarsaihan D. "Epigenetic mechanisms in inflammation." J Dent Res 90: 9–17 (2011)

Belfort MB, Rifas-Shiman SL, Kleinman KP, Guthrie LB, Bellinger DC, Taveras EM, Gillman MW, and Oken E. "Infant feeding and childhood cognition at ages 3 and 7 years: Effects of breastfeeding duration and exclusivity." JAMA Pediatr 167: 836–844 (2013)

Blasbalg TL, Hibbeln JR, Ramsden CE, Majchrzak SF, and Rawlings RR. "Changes in consumption of omega-3 and omega-6 fatty acids in the United States during the 20th century." Am J Clin Nutr 93: 950–962 (2011)

Chalon S, Vancassel S, Zimmer L, Guilloteau D, and Durand G. "Polyunsaturated fatty acids and cerebral function: focus on monoaminergic neurotransmission." Lipids 36: 937–944 (2001)

Chong S and Whitelaw E. "Epigenetic germline inheritance." Curr Opin Genet Dev 14: 692–696 (2004)

Ding Y, Li J, Liu S, Zhang L, Xiao H, Li J, Chen H, Petersen RB, Huang K, and Zheng L. "DNA hypomethylation of inflammation-associated genes in adipose tissue of female mice after multigenerational high fat diet feeding." Int J Obes 38: 198–204 (2014)

Grayson DS, Kroenke CD, Neuringer M, and Fair DA. "Dietary omega-3 fatty acids modulate large-scale systems organization in the rhesus macaque brain." J Neurosci 34: 2065–2074 (2014)

Hanbauer I, Rivero-Covelo I, Maloku E, Baca A, Hu Q, Hibbeln JR, and Davis JM. "The decrease of n-3 fatty acid energy percentage in an equicaloric diet fed to B6C3Fe mice for three generations elicits obesity." Cardiovasc Psychiatry Neurol 2009: 867041 (2009)

Massiera F, Saint-Marc P, Seydoux J, Murata T, Kobayashi T, Narumiya S, Guesnet P, Amri EZ, Negrel R, and Ailhaud G. "Arachidonic acid and prostacyclin signaling promote adipose tissue development: a human health concern?" J Lipid Res 44: 271–279 (2003)

Massiera F, Barbry p, Guesnet P, Joly A, Luquet S, Moreihon-Brest C, Moshen-Kanson T, Amri EZ, and Ailhaud G. "A western-like diet is sufficient to induce a gradual enhancement in fat mass over generations." J Lipid Res 51: 2352–2361 (2010)

Muhlauser BS, Cook-Johnson R, James M, Miljkovic D, Duthoit E, and Gibson R. "Opposing effects of omega-3 and omega-6 long polyunsaturated fatty acids on the expression of lipogenic genes in omental and retroperitoneal adipose depots in the rat." J Nutr Metabol 2010: 1–9 (2010)

Mulhausler BS and Ailhaud GP. "Omega-6 polyunsaturated fatty acid and the early origins of obesity." Curr Opin Endocrinol Diabetes Obes 20: 55–61 (2013)

Olshansky SJ, Passaro DJ, Hershow RC, Layden J, Carnes BA, Brody J, Hayflick L, Butler RN, Allison DB, and Ludwig DS. "A potential decline in life expectancy in the United States in the 21st century." N Engl J Med 352: 1138–1145 (2005)

Ravelli AC, van Der Meulen JH, Osmond C, Barker DJ, and Bleker OP. "Obesity at the age of 50 y in men and women exposed to famine prenatally." Am J Clin Nutr 70: 811–816 (1999)

Roseboom TJ, van der Meulen JH, Ravelli AC, Osmond C, Barker DJ, and Bleker OP. "Effects of prenatal exposure to the Dutch famine on adult disease in later life: an overview." Mol Cell Endocrinol 185: 93–98 (2001)

Roseboom TJ and Watson ED. "The next generation of disease risk: are the effects of prenatal nutrition transmitted across generations?" Placenta 33: e40–e44 (2012)

Painter RC, de Rooij SR, Bossuyt PM, Simmers TA, Osmond C, Barker DJ, Bleker OP, and Roseboom TJ. "Early onset of coronary artery disease after prenatal exposure to the Dutch famine." Am J Clin Nutr 84: 322–327 (2006)

Tollefsbol T (ed). *Epigenetics in Human Disease*. Academic Press. New York, NY (2012)

Tollefsbol TO. "Dietary epigenetics in cancer and aging." Cancer Treat Res 159: 257–267 (2014)

CHAPTER 14: RECLAIMING OUR GENETIC FUTURE

Bayarsaihan D. "Epigenetic mechanisms in inflammation." J Dent Res 90: 9–17 (2011)

Crane PK, Walker R, Hubbard RA, Li G, Nathan DM, Zheng H, Haneuse S, Craft S, Montine TJ, Kahn SE, McCormick W, McCurry SM, Bowen JD, and Larson EB. "Glucose levels and risk of dementia." N Engl J Med 369: 540–548 (2013)

James BD, Leurgans SE, Hebert LE, Scherr PA, Yaffe K, and Bennett DA. "Contribution of Alzheimer disease to mortality in the United States." Neurology 82: 1045–1050 (2014)

Goldman DP, Cutler D, Rowe JW, Michaud P, Sullivan, J, Peneva K, and Olshansky SJ. "Substantial health and economic returns from delayed aging may warrant a new focus for medical research." Health Affairs 32: 1698–1705 (2013)

Hanbauer I, Rivero-Covelo I, Maloku E, Baca A, Hu Q, Hibbeln JR, and Davis JM. "The decrease of n-3 fatty acid energy percentage in an equicaloric diet fed to B6C3Fe mice for three generations elicits obesity." Cardiovasc Psychiatry Neurol 2009: 867041 (2009)

Holmes C. "Review: systemic inflammation and Alzheimer's disease." Neuropathol Appl Neurobiol 39: 51–68 (2013)

Sears B. *The Zone*. Regan Books. New York, NY (1995)

Sears B. *Mastering the Zone*. Regan Books. New York, NY (1997)

Sears B. *The Anti-Aging Zone*. Regan Books. New York, NY (1999)

Sears B. *The OmegaRx Zone*. Regan Books. New York, NY (2002)

Sears B. *The Anti-Inflammation Zone*. Regan Books. New York, NY (2005)

Sears B. *Toxic Fat*. Thomas Nelson. Nashville, TN (2008)

Spite M, Claria J, and Serhan CN. "Resolvins, specialized proresolving lipid mediators and their potential roles in metabolic diseases." Cell Metabolism 19: 21–36 (2014)

Tollefsbol T (ed). *Epigenetics in Human Disease*. Academic Press. New York, NY (2012)

Tollesfsbol TO. "Dietary epigenetics in cancer and aging." Cancer Treat Res 159: 257–267 (2014)

APPENDIX B. THE SCIENCE OF DIET-INDUCED INFLAMMATION

Appel S, Mirakaj V, Bringmann A, Weck MM, Grunebach F, and Brossart P. "PPAR-gamma agonists inhibit toll-like receptor-mediated activation of dendritic cells via the MAP kinase and NF-kappaB pathways." Blood 106: 3888–3894 (2005)

Arbo I, Halle C, Malik D, Brattbakk HR, and Johansen B. "Insulin induces fatty acid desaturase expression in human monocytes." Scand J Clin Lab Invest 71: 330–339 (2011)

Blasbalg TL, Hibbeln JR, Ramsden CE, Majchrzak SF, and Rawlings RR. "Changes in consumption of omega-3 and omega-6 fatty acids in the United States during the 20th century." Am J Clin Nutr 93: 950–962 (2011)

Brenner RR. "Hormonal modulation of delta-6 and delta-5 desaturases: case of diabetes." Prostaglandins Leukot Essent Fatty Acids 68: 151–162 (2003)

Chakrabarti SK, Cole BK, Wen Y, Keller SR, and Nadler JL. "12/15-lipoxygenase products induce inflammation and impair insulin signaling in 3T3-L1 adipocytes." Obesity 17: 1657–1663 (2009)

Chapkin RS, McMurray DN, Davidson LA, Patil BS, Fan YY, and Lupton JR. "Bioactive dietary long-chain fatty acids: emerging mechanisms of action." Br J Nutr 100: 1152–1157 (2008)

Chen CT, Liu Z, Ouellet M, Calon F, and Bazinet RP. "Rapid beta-oxidation of eicosapentaenoic acid in mouse brain: an in situ study." Prostaglandins Leukot Essent Fatty Acids 80: 157–163 (2009)

Chen CT, Liu Z, and Bazinet RP. "Rapid de-esterification and loss of eicosapentaenoic acid from rat brain phospholipids: an intracerebroventricular study." J Neurochem 116: 363–373 (2011)

el Boustani S, Causse JE, Descomps B, Monnier L, Mendy F, and Crastes de Paulet A. "Direct in vivo characterization of delta 5 desaturase activity in humans by deuterium labeling: effect of insulin." Metabolism 38: 315–321 (1989)

Farooqui AA. "n-3 fatty acid-derived lipid mediators in the brain: new weapons against oxidative stress and inflammation." Curr Med Chem 19: 532–543 (2012)

Harris WS, Pottala JV, Varvel SA, Borowski JJ, Ward JN, and McConnell JP. "Erythrocyte omega-3 fatty acids increase and linoleic acid decreases with age: observations from 160,000 patients." Prostaglandins Leukot Essent Fatty Acids 88: 257–263 (2013)

Kawabata T, Hirota S, Hirayama T, Adachi N, Hagiwara C, Iwama N, Kamachi K, Araki E, Kawashima H, and Kiso Y. "Age-related changes of dietary intake and blood eicosapentaenoic acid, docosahexaenoic acid, and arachidonic acid levels in Japanese men and women." Prostaglandins Leukot Essent Fatty Acids 84: 131–137 (2011)

Li Q, Wang M, Tan L, Wang C, Ma J, Li N, Li Y, Xu G, and Li J. "Docosahexaenoic acid changes lipid composition and interleukin-2 receptor signaling in membrane rafts." J Lipid Res 46: 1904–1913 (2005)

Martinez-Clemente M, Claria J, and Titos E. "The 5-lipoxygenase/leukotriene pathway in obesity, insulin resistance, and fatty liver disease." Curr Opin Clin Nutr Metab Care 14: 347–353 (2011)

Mori TA, Burke V, Puddey IB, Watts GF, O'Neal DN, Best JD, and Beilin LJ. "Purified eicosapentaenoic and docosahexaenoic acids have differential effects on serum lipids and lipoproteins, LDL particle size, glucose, and insulin in mildly hyperlipidemic men." Am J Clin Nutr 71: 1085–1094 (2000)

Pelikanova T, Kohout M, Base J, Stefka Z, Kovar J, Kazdova L, and Valek J. "Effect of acute hyperinsulinemia on fatty acid composition of serum lipids in non-insulin-dependent diabetics and healthy men." Clin Chim Acta 203: 329–337 (1991)

Plourde M and Cunnane SC. "Extremely limited synthesis of long chain polyunsaturates in adults: implications for their dietary essentiality and use as supplements." Appl Physiol Nutr Metab 32: 619–634 (2007)

Rahman I, Biswas SK, and Kirkham PA. "Regulation of inflammation and redox signaling by dietary polyphenols." Biochem Pharmacol 72: 1439–1452 (2006)

Rizzo AM, Montorfano G, Negroni M, Adorni L, Berselli P, Corsetto P, Wahle K, and Berra B. "A rapid method for determining arachidonic: eicosapentaenoic acid ratios in whole blood lipids: correlation with erythrocyte membrane ratios and validation in a large Italian population of various ages and pathologies." Lipids Health Dis 9: 7 (2010)

Sanchez-Galan E, Gomez-Hernandez A, Vidal C, Martin-Ventura JL, Blanco-Colio LM, Munoz-Garcia B, Ortega L, Egido J, and Tunon J. "Leukotriene B4 enhances the activity of nuclear factor-kappaB pathway through BLT1 and BLT2 receptors in atherosclerosis." Cardiovasc Res 81: 216–225 (2009)

Scapagnini G, Vasto S, Sonya V, Abraham NG, Nader AG, Caruso C, Calogero C, Zella D, and Fabio G. "Modulation of Nrf2/ARE pathway by food polyphenols: a nutritional neuroprotective strategy for cognitive and neurodegenerative disorders." Mol Neurobiol 44: 192–201 (2011)

Schmitz G and Ecker J. "The opposing effect of n-3 and n-6 fatty acids." Prog Lipid Res 47: 147–155 (2008)

Sears, B. The Zone. Regan Books. New York, NY (1995)

Sears, B. The Anti-Aging Zone. Regan Books. New York, NY (1999)

Sears, B. The OmegaRx Zone. Regan Books. New York, NY (2002)

Sears, B. The Anti-Inflammation Zone. Regan Books. New York, NY (2005)

Sears, B. Toxic Fat. Thomas Nelson. Nashville, TN. (2008)

Sears B and Ricordi C. "Role of fatty acids and polyphenols in inflammatory gene transcription and their impact on obesity, metabolic syndrome and diabetes." Eur Rev Med Pharmacol Sci 16: 1137–1154 (2012)

Sears DD, Miles PD, Chapman J, Ofrecio JM, Almazan F, Thapar D, and Miller YI. "12/15-lipoxygenase is required for the early onset of high fat diet-induced adipose tissue inflammation and insulin resistance in mice." PLoS ONE 4: e7250 (2009)

Stillwell W and Wassall SR. "Docosahexaenoic acid: membrane properties of a unique fatty acid." Chem Phys Lipids 126: 1–27 (2003)

Tall AR. "C-reactive protein reassessed." N Engl J Med 350: 1450–1452 (2004)

Umhau JC, Zhou W, Carson RE, Rapoport SI, Polozova A, Demar J, Hussein N, Bhattacharjee AK, Ma K, Esposito G, Majchrzak S, Herscovitch P, Eckelman WC, Kurdziel KA, and Salem N. "Imaging incorporation of circulating docosahexaenoic acid into the human brain using positron emission tomography." J Lipid Res 50: 1259–1268 (2009)

Zhang MJ and Spite M. "Resolvins: anti-inflammatory and proresolving mediators derived from omega-3 polyunsaturated fatty acids." Annu Rev Nutr 32: 203–227 (2012)

APPENDIX C. INFLAMMATORY AND OBESITY

Ailhaud G, Guesnet P, and Cunnane SC. "An emerging risk factor for obesity: does disequilibrium of polyunsaturated fatty acid metabolism contribute to excessive adipose tissue development?" Br J Nutr 100: 461–470 (2008)

Ailhaud G. "Omega-6 fatty acids and excessive adipose tissue development." World Rev Nutr Diet 98: 51–61 (2008)

Alvheim AR, Malde MK, Osei-Hyiaman D, Lin YH, Pawlosky RJ, Madsen L, Kristiansen K, Froyland L, and Hibbeln JR. "Dietary linoleic acid elevates endogenous 2-AG and anandamide and induces obesity." Obesity 10: 1984–1994 (2012)

Alvheim AR, Torstensen BE, Lin YH, Lillefosse HH, Lock EJ, Madsen L, Froyland L, Hibbeln JR, and Malde MK. "Dietary linoleic acid elevates the endocannabinoids 2-AG and anandamide and promotes weight gain in mice fed a low fat diet." Lipids 49: 59–69 (2014)

Batterham RL, Heffron H, Kapoor S, Chivers JE, Chandarana K, Herzon H, le Roux CW, Thomas EL, Bell JD, and Withers DJ. "Critical role for peptide YY in protein-mediated satiation and body-weight regulation." Cell Metabol 4: 223–233 (2006)

Benhamed F, Poupeau A, and Postic C. "The transcription factor ChREBP: a key modulator of insulin sensitivity?" Med Sci 29: 765–771 (2013)

Beglinger C and Degen L. "Gastrointestinal satiety signals in humans—physiologic roles for GLP-1 and PYY?" Physiol Behav 89: 460–464 (2006)

Berg JM, Tymoczko JL, and Stryer L. Biochemistry, 5th edition. W.H. Freeman. New York, NY (2002)

Bilsborough S and Mann N. "A review of issues of dietary protein intake in humans." Int J Sport Nutr Exerc Metab 16: 129–152 (2006)

Buckland G. Bach A. and Serra-Majem L. "Obesity and the Mediterranean diet: a systematic review of observational and intervention studies." Obes Rev 9: 582–593 (2008)

Cai D. "Neuroinflammation and neurodegeneration in overnutrition-induced diseases." Trends Endocrinol Metab 24: 40–47 (2013)

Chaudhri OB, Field BC, and Bloom SR. "Gastrointestinal satiety signals." Int J Obes 7: S28–31 (2008)

Claria J, Dalli J, Yacoubian S, Gao F, and Serhan CN. "Resolvin D1 and resolvin D2 govern local inflammatory tone in obese fat." J Immunology 189: 2597–2605 (2012)

Cole BK, Lieb DC, Dobrian AD, and Nadler JL. "12- and -15 lipoxygenases in adipose tissue inflammation." Prostaglandins and Other Lipid Mediators 105: 84–92 (2013)

Czech MP, Tencerova M, Pedersen DJ, and Aouadi M. "Insulin signaling mechanisms for triacylglycerol storage." Diabetologia 56: 949–964 (2013)

Dentin R, Denechaud P-D, Benhamed F, Girad J, and Postic C. "Hepatic gene regulation by glucose and polyunsaturated fatty acids: a role for ChREBP." J Nutr 136: 1145–1149 (2006)

Dockray GJ. "Cholecystokinin." Curr Opin Endocrinol Diabetes Obes 19: 8–12 (2012)

Ebbeling CB, Swain JF, Feldman HA, Wong WW, Hachey DL, Garcia-Lago E, and Ludwig DS. "Effects of dietary composition on energy expenditure during weight-loss maintenance." JAMA 307: 2627–2634 (2012)

Flachs P, Horakova O, Brauner P, Rossmeisl M, Pecina P, Franssen-van Hal N, Ruzickova J, Sponarova J, Drahota Z, Vlcek C, Keijer J, Houstek J, and Kopecky J. "Poly-unsaturated fatty acids of marine origin upregulate mitochondrial biogenesis and induce beta-oxidation in white fat." Diabetologia 48: 2365–2375 (2005)

Gonzalex-Periz A, Horrillo R, Ferre N, Gronert K, Dong B, Moran-Salvador E, Titos E, Martinez-Clemente M, Lopez-Parra M, Arroyo V, and Claria J. "Obesity-induced insulin resistance and hepatic steatosis are alleviated by omega-3 fatty acids: a role for resolvins and protectins." FASEB J 23: 1946–1957 (2009)

Gregor MF and Hotamisligil GS. "Inflammatory mechanisms in obesity." Ann Rev Immunol 29: 415–445 (2011)

Hanbauer I, Rivero-Covelo I, Maloku E, Baca A, Hu Q, Hibbeln JR, and Davis JM. "The decrease of n-3 fatty acid energy percentage in an equicaloric diet fed to B6C3Fe mice for three generations elicits obesity." Cardiovasc Psychiatry Neurol 2009: 867041 (2009)

Itariu BK, Zeyda M, Hochbrugger EE, Neuhofer A, Prager G, Schindler K; Bohdjalian A, Mascher D, Vangala S, Schranz M, Krebs M, Bischof MG, and Stulnig TM. "Long-chain n-3 PUFAs reduce adipose tissue and systemic inflammation in severely obese nondiabetic patients: a randomized controlled trial." Am J Clin Nutr 96: 1137–1149 (2012)

Jin C and Flavell RA. "Innate sensors of pathogen and stress: linking inflammation to obesity." J Allergy Clin Immunol 132: 287–294 (2013)

Jornayvaz FR, Jurczak MJ, Lee HY, Birkenfeld AL, Frederick DW, Zhang D, Zhang XM, Samuel VT, and Shulman GI. "A high-fat, ketogenic diet causes hepatic insulin resistance in mice, despite increasing energy expenditure and preventing weight gain." Am J Physiol Endocrinol Metab. 299: E808–15 (2010)

Kim J, Li Y, and Watkins BA. "Fat to treat fat: emerging relationship between dietary PUFA, endocannabinoids, and obesity." Prostaglandins Other Lipid Mediators 105: 32–41 (2013)

Kirkham TC. "Endocannabinoids and the non-homeostatic control of appetite." Curr Top Behav Neurosci 1: 231–253 (2009)

Lafontan M and Langin D. "Lipolysis and lipid mobilization in human adipose tissue." Prog Lipid Res. 48: 275–297 (2009)

le Roux CW, Batterham RL, Aylwin SJLB, Patterson, Borg Cm, Wynee KJ, Kent A, Vincent RP, Gardiner J, Ghati MA, and Bloom SR. "Attenuated peptide YY release in-obese subjects is associated with reduced satiety." Endocrinology 147: 3–8 (2006)

Lennerz BS, Alsop DC, Holsen LM, Stern E, Rojas R, Ebbeling CB, Goldstein JM, and Ludwig DS. "Effects of dietary glycemic index on brain regions related to reward and craving in men." Am J Clin Nutr 98: 641–647 (2013)

Lumrn CN and Saltiel AR. "Inflammatory links between obesity and metabolic disease." J Clin Invest 121: 2111–2117 (2011)

Massiera F, Saint-Marc P, Seydoux J, Murata T, Kobayashi T, Narumiya S, Guesnet P, Amri EZ, Negrel R, and Ailhaud G. "Arachidonic acid and prostacyclin signaling promote adipose tissue development: a human health concern?" J Lipid Res 44: 271–279 (2003)

Murphy KG and Bloom SR. "Gut hormones and the regulation of energy homeostatsis." Nature 444: 854–858 (2006)

Neuhofer A, Zeyda M, Mascher D, Itariu BK, Murano I, Leitner L, Hochbrugger EE,

Fraisl P, Cinti S, Serhan CN, and Stulnig TM. "Impaired local production of prore-solving lipid mediators in obesity and 17-HDHA as a potential treatment for obesity-associated inflammation." Diabetes 62: 1945–1956 (2013)

Padwal RS, Pajewski NM, Allison DB, and Sharma AM. "Using the Edmonton obesity staging system to predict mortality in a population-representative cohort of people with overweight and obesity." CMAJ 183: E1059–1066 (2011)

Porte D, Baskin DG, and Schwartz MW. "Leptin and insulin action in the central nervous system." Nutr Rev 60: S20–9 (2002)

Parks BW, Nam E, Org E, Kostem E, Norheim F, Hui ST, Pan C, Civelek M, Rau CD, Bennett BJ, Mehrabian M, Ursell LK, He A, Castellani LW, Zinker B, Kirby M, Drake TA, Drevon CA, Knight R, Gargalovic P, Kirchgessner T, Eskin E, and Lusis AJ. "Genetic control of obesity and gut microbiota composition in response to high-fat, high-sucrose diet in mice." Cell Metab 17: 141–152 (2013)

Postic C, Dentin R, Denechaud PD, and Girard J. "ChREBP, a transcriptional regulator of glucose and lipid metabolism." Annu Rev Nutr 27: 179–192 (2007)

Ramel PD, Bandarra N, Kiely M, Marinez JA, and Thorsdottir I. "A diet rich in long chain omega-3 fatty acids modulates satiety in overweight and obese volunteers during weight loss." Appetite 51: 676–680 (2008)

Ribet C, Montastier E, Valle C, Bezaire V, Mazzucotelli A, Mairal A, Viguerie N, and Langin D. "Peroxisome proliferator-activated receptor-alpha control of lipid and glucose metabolism in human white adipocytes." Endocrinology 151: 123–133 (2010)

Reilly SM and Satiel AR. "Obesity: A complex role for adipose tissue macrophages." Nat Rev Endocrin 10: 193–194 (2014)

Sadur CN and Eckel RH. "Insulin stimulation of adipose tissue lipoprotein lipase. Use of the euglycemic clamp technique." J Clin Invest 69: 1119–1125 (1982)

Saltzman E and Karl JP. "Nutrient deficiencies after gastric bypass surgery." Annu Rev Nutr 33: 183–203 (2013)

Schwartz MW and Morton GJ. "Keeping hunger at bay." Nature 418: 595–597 (2002)

Sears B. *Toxic Fat*. Thomas Nelson. Nashville, TN. (2008)

Soria-Gómez E, Bellocchio L, Reguero L, Lepousez G, Martin C, Bendahmane M, Ruehle S, Remmers F, Desprez T, Matias I, Wiesner T, Cannich A, Nissant A, Wadleigh A, Pape HC, Chiarlone AP, Quarta C, Verrier D, Vincent P, Massa F, Lutz B, Guzmán M, Gurden H, Ferreira G, Lledo PM, Grandes P, and Marsicano G. "The endocannabinoid system controls food intake via olfactory processes." Nat Neurosci 17: 407–415 (2014)

Storlien L, Oakes ND, and Kelley DE. "Metabolic flexibility." Proc Nutr Soc 63: 363–368 (2004)

Sumithran P, Prendergast LA, Delbridge E, Purcell K, Shulkes A, Kriketos A, and Proietto J. "Long-term persistence of hormonal adaptations to weight loss." N Engl J Med 365: 1597–1604 (2011)

Thaler JP and Schwartz MW. "Minireview: Inflammation and obesity pathogenesis: the hypothalamus heats up." Endocrinology 151: 4109–4115 (2010)

Thomas JG, Bond DS, Phelan S, Hill JO, and Wing RR. "Weight-loss maintenance for 10 years in the National Weight Control Registry." Am J Prev Med 46: 17–23 (2014)

Titos E and Claria J. "Omega-3-derived mediators counteract obesity-induced adipose tissue inflammation." Prostaglandins Other Lipid Mediators 107: 77–84 (2013)

Todoric J, Loffler M, Huber J, Bilban M, Reimers M, Kadl A, Zeyda M, Waldhausl W, and Stulnig TM. "Adipose tissue inflammation induced by high-fat diet in obese diabetic mice is prevented by n-3 polyunsaturated fatty acids." Diabetologia 49: 2109–2119 (2006)

Unger RH. "Lipotoxic diseases." Annu Rev Med 53: 319–336 (2002)

Veldhorst M, Smeets A, Soenen S, Hochstenbach-Waelen A, Hursel R, Diepvens K, Lejeune M, Luscombe-Marsh N, and Westerterp-Plantenga M. "Protein-induced satiety: effects and mechanisms of different proteins." Physiol Behav 94: 300–307 (2008)

Vincent RP and le Roux CW. "Changes in gut hormones after bariatric surgery." Clin Endocrinol 69: 173–179 (2008)

APPENDIX D. INFLAMMATION AND CHRONIC DISEASE

Arbo I, Halle C, Malik D, Brattbakk HR, and Johansen B. "Insulin induces fatty acid desaturase expression in human monocytes."Scand J Clin Lab Invest 71: 330–339 (2011)

Baylin A and Campos H. "Arachidonic acid in adipose tissue is associated with nonfatal acute myocardial infarction in the central valley of Costa Rica." J Nutr. 134: 3095–3099 (2004)

Brenner RR. "Hormonal modulation of delta-6 and delta-5 desaturases: case of diabetes." Prostaglandins Leukot Essent Fatty Acids 68: 151–162 (2003)

Cawood AL, Ding R, Napper FL, Young RH, Williams JA, Ward MJ, Gudmundsen O, Vige R, Payne SP, Ye S, Shearman CP, Gallagher PJ, Grimble RF, and Calder PC. "Eicosapentaenoic acid (EPA) from highly concentrated n-3 fatty acid ethyl esters is incorporated into advanced atherosclerotic plaques and higher plaque EPA is associated with decreased plaque inflammation and increased stability." Atherosclerosis 212: 252–259 (2010)

el Boustani S, Causse JE, Descomps B, Monnier L, Mendy F, and Crastes de Paulet A. "Direct in vivo characterization of delta 5 desaturase activity in humans by deuterium labeling: effect of insulin." Metabolism 38: 315–321 (1989)

Glass CK and Olefsky JM. "Inflammation and lipid signaling in the etiology of insulin resistance." Cell Metab. 15: 635–645 (2012)

Greenhough A, Smartt HJ, Moore AE, Roberts HR, Williams AC, Paraskeva C, and Kaidi A. "The COX-2/PGE2 pathway: key roles in the hallmarks of cancer and adaptation to the tumour microenvironment." Carcinogenesis 30: 377–386 (2009)

Greene ER, Huang S, Serhan CN, and Panigrahy D. "Regulation of inflammation in cancer by eicosanoids." Prostaglandins and Other Lipid Mediators 96: 27–36 (2011)

Holvoet P. "Oxidized LDL and coronary heart disease." Acta Cardiol 59: 479–484 (2004)

Hotamisligil GS, Arner P, Caro JF, Atkinson RL, and Spiegelman BM. "Increased adipose tissue expression of tumor necrosis factor-alpha in human obesity and insulin resistance." J Clin Invest 95: 2409–2415 (1995)

Ishigaki Y, Oka Y, and Katagiri H. "Circulating oxidized LDL: a biomarker and a pathogenic factor." Curr Opin Lipidol 20: 363–369 (2009)

Jornayvaz FR, Jurczak MJ, Lee HY, Birkenfeld AL, Frederick DW, Zhang D, Zhang XM, Samuel VT, and Shulman GI. "A high-fat, ketogenic diet causes hepatic insulin resistance in mice, despite increasing energy expenditure and preventing weight gain." Am J Physiol Endocrinol Metab 299: E808–15 (2010)

Joslin Diabetes Reseach Center. www.joslin.org/docs/Nutrition_Guideline_Graded.pdfEPIC and Diabetes (2007)

Kratsovnik E, Bromberg Y, Sperling O, and Zoref-Shani E. "Oxidative stress activates transcription factor NF-kB-mediated protective signaling in primary rat neuronal cultures." J Mol Neurosci 26: 27–32 (2005)

Krishnamoorthy S and Honn KV. "Eicosanoids in tumor progression and metastasis." Subcell Biochem 49: 145–168 (2008)

Leaf C. The Truth in Small Doses: Why We're Losing the War on Cancer-and How to Win It. Simon and Shuster. New York, NY (2013)

Li N and Karin M. "Is NF-kappaB the sensor of oxidative stress?" FASEB J 13: 1137–1143 (1999)

Maruyama C, Imamura K, and Teramoto T. "Assessment of LDL particle size by triglyceride/HDL-cholesterol ratio in non-diabetic, healthy subjects without prominent hyperlipidemia." J Atheroscler Thromb 10: 186–91 (2003)

McLaughlin T, Reaven G, Abbasi F, Lamendola C, Saad M, Waters D, Simon J, and Krauss RM. "Is there a simple way to identify insulin-resistant individuals at increased risk of cardiovascular disease?" Am J Cardiol 96: 399–404 (2005)

Meisinger C, Baumert J, Khuseyinova N, Lowel H, and Koenig W. "Plasma oxidized low-density lipoprotein, a strong predictor for acute coronary heart disease events in apparently healthy, middle-aged men from the general population." Circulation 112: 651–657 (2005)

Miller BS and Yee D. "Type I insulin-like growth factor receptor as a therapeutic target in cancer." Cancer Res 65: 10123–10137 (2005)

Nazaryan A. "Getting Cancer Wrong." Newsweek. March 20, 2014 (2014)

Nielsen MS, Gronholdt M-L, Vyberg M, Overvad K, Andreasen A, Due K-M, and Schmidt EB. "Adipose tissue arachidonic acid content is associated with expression of 5-lipoxygenase in atherosclerotic plaques." Lipids in Health and Dis 12: 7 (2013)

Pelikanova T, Kohout M, Base J, Stefka Z, Kovar J, Kazdova L, and Valek J. "Effect of acute hyperinsulinemia on fatty acid composition of serum lipids in non-insulin-dependent diabetics and healthy men." Clin Chim Acta 203: 329–337 (1991)

Rahman I, Gilmour PS, Jimenez LA, and MacNee W. "Oxidative stress and TNF-alpha induce histone acetylation and NF-kappaB/AP-1 activation in alveolar epithelial cells: potential mechanism in gene transcription in lung inflammation." Mol Cell Biochem 235: 239–248 (2002)

Rhee JW, Lee KW, Kim D, Lee Y, Jeon OH, Kwon HJ, and Kim DS. "NF-kappaB-dependent regulation of matrix metalloproteinase-9 gene expression by lipopolysaccharide in a macrophage cell line RAW 264.7." J Biochem Mol Biol 40: 88–94 (2007)

Sears B. The Anti-inflammation Zone. Regan Books. New York, NY (2005)

Sears B. Toxic Fat. Thomas Nelson. Nashville, TN (2008)

Tabues G. "Prosperity's Plague." Science 325: 256–260 (2009)

Terrando N, Gomez-Galan M, Yang T, Carlstrom M, Gustavsson D, Harding RE, Lindskog M, and Eriksson LI. "Asprin-triggered resolvin D1 prevent surgery-induced cognitive decline." FASEB J 27: 3564–3571 (2013)

Thies F, Garry JM, Yaqoob P, Rerkasem K, Williams J, Shearman CP, Gallagher PJ, Calder PC, and Grimble RF. "Association of n-3 polyunsaturated fatty acids with stability of atherosclerotic plaques: a randomised controlled trial." Lancet. 361: 477–485 (2003)

Wassink AM, Van Der Graaf Y, Soedamah-Muthu SS, Spiering W, and Visseren FL. "Metabolic syndrome and incidence of type 2 diabetes in patients with manifest vascular disease." Diab Vasc Dis Res 5: 114–122 (2008)

Wierzbicki AS, Purdon SD, Hardman TC, Kulasegaram R, and Peters BS. "HIV lipodystrophy and its metabolic consequences: implications for clinical practice." Curr Med Res Opin 24: 609–624 (2008)

Williams ES, Baylin A, and Campos H. "Adipose tissue arachidonic acid and the metabolic syndrome in Costa Rican adults." Clin Nutr 26: 474–482 (2007)

Zhang X, Zhang G, Zhang H, Karin M, Bai H, and Cai D. "Hypothalamic IKKbeta/NF-kappaB and ER stress link overnutrition to energy imbalance and obesity." Cell 135: 61–73 (2008)

APPENDIX E. INFLAMMATION AND AGING

Ambati J, Atkinson JP, and Gelfand BD. "Immunology of age-related macular degeneration." Nat Rev Immunol 13: 438–451 (2013)

Bjorntorp P. "Hormonal control of regional fat distribution." Hum Reprod 12 Suppl 1: 21–25 (1997)

Borg M, Brincat S, Camilleri G, Schembri-Wismayer P, Brincat M, and Calleja-Agius J. "The role of cytokines in skin aging." Climacteric 16: 514–521 (2013)

Casado-Díaz A, Santiago-Mora R, Dorado G, and Quesada-Gómez JM. "The omega-6 arachidonic fatty acid, but not the omega-3 fatty acids, inhibits osteoblastogenesis and induces adipogenesis of human mesenchymal stem cells: potential implication in osteoporosis." Osteoporos Int 24: 1647–1661 (2013)

Gao L, Faibish D, Fredman G, Herrera BS, Chiang N, Serhan CN, Van Dyke TE, and Gyurko R. "Resolvin E1 and chemokine-like receptor 1 mediate bone preservation." J Immunol 190: 689–694 (2013)

Garza LA, Liu Y, Yang Z, Alagesan B, Lawson JA, Norberg SM, Loy DE, Zhao T, Blatt HB, Stanton DC, Carrasco L, Ahluwalia G, Fischer SM, FitzGerald GA, and Cotsarelis G. "Prostaglandin D2 inhibits hair growth and is elevated in bald scalp of men with androgenetic alopecia." Sci Transl Med. 4: 126ra34 (2012)

Georgiou T, Neokleous A, Nikolaou D, and Sears B. "Pilot study for treating dry age-related macular degeneration (AMD) with high-dose omega-3 fatty acids." Pharma-Nutrition 2: 8–11 (2014)

Guertin DA and Sabatini DM. "Defining the role of mTOR in cancer." Cancer Cell 12: 9–22 (2007)

Jenkins G. "Molecular mechanisms of skin ageing." Mech Ageing Dev 123: 801–810 (2002)

Li F, Yin Y, Tan B, Kong X, and Wu G. "Leucine nutrition in animals and humans: mTOR signaling and beyond." Amino Acids 41: 1185–1193 (2011)

Nieves A and Garza LA. "Does prostaglandin D2 hold the cure to male pattern baldness?" Exp Dermatol. 23: 224–227 (2014)

Norton LE, Wilson GJ, Layman DK, Moulton CJ, and Garlick PJ. "Leucine content of dietary proteins is a determinant of postprandial skeletal muscle protein synthesis in adult rats." Nutr Metab 20: 67 (2012)

Rahman I, Biswas SK, and Kirkham PA. "Regulation of inflammation and redox signaling by dietary polyphenols." Biochem Pharmacol 72: 1439–1452 (2006)

Scapagnini G, Vasto S, Abraham NG, Caruso C, Zella D, and Fabio G. "Modulation of Nrf2/ARE pathway by food polyphenols: a nutritional neuroprotective strategy for cognitive and neurodegenerative disorders." Mol Neurobiol 44: 192–201 (2011)

Sears, B. *The Anti-Aging Zone*. Regan Books. New York, NY (1999)

Shi Y, Luo LF, Liu XM, Zhou Q, Xu SZ, and Lei TC. "Premature graying as a consequence of compromised antioxidant activity in hair bulb melanocytes and their precursors." PLoS One9: e93589 (2014)

Shinto L, Marracci G, Baldauf-Wagner S, Strehlow A, Yadav V, Stuber L, and Bourdette D. "Omega-3 fatty acid supplementation decreases matrix metalloproteinase-9 production in relapsing-remitting multiple sclerosis." Prostaglandins Leukot Essent Fatty Acids 80: 131–136 (2009)

Tanaka K, Asamitsu K, Uranishi H, Iddamalgoda A, Ito K, Kojima H, and Okamoto T. "Protecting skin photoaging by NF-kappaB inhibitor." Curr Drug Metab11: 431–435 (2010)

Wang F, Mullican SE, DiSpirito JR, Peed LC, and Lazar MA. "Lipoatrophy and severe metabolic disturbance in mice with fat-specific deletion of PPARγ." Proc Natl Acad Sci U S A110: 18656–18661 (2013)

APPENDIX F. MARKERS OF WELLNESS

Bierhaus A, Stern DM, and Nawroth PP. "RAGE in inflammation: a new therapeutic target?" Curr Opin Investig Drugs 7: 985–991 (2006)

Carson AP, Fox CS, McGuire DK, Levitan EB, Laclaustra M, Mann DM, and Muntner P. "Low hemoglobin A1c and risk of all-cause mortality among US adults without diabetes." Circ Cardiovasc Qual Outcomes 3: 661–667 (2010)

Campbell B, Badrick T, Flatman R, and Kanowski D. "Limited clinical utility of high-sensitivity plasma C-reactive protein assays." Ann Clin Biochem39: 85–88 (2002)

Campbell B, Flatman R, Badrick T, and Kanowski D. "Problems with high-sensitivity C-reactive protein." Clin Chem 49: 201 (2003)

Endres S, Ghorbani R, Kelley VE, Georgilis K, Lonnemann G, van der Meer JW, Cannon JG, Rogers TS, Klempner MS, Weber PC, Schafter EJ, Wolff SM, and Dinarello CA. "The effect of dietary supplementation with n-3 polyunsaturated fatty acids on the synthesis of interleukin-1 and tumor necrosis factor by mononuclear cells." N Engl J Med 320: 265–271 (1989)

Harris WS, Pottala JV, Varvel SA, Borowski JJ, Ward JN, and McConnell JP. "Erythrocyte omega-3 fatty acids increase and linoleic acid decreases with age: observations from 160,000 patients." Prostaglandins Leukot Essent Fatty Acids. 88: 257–263 (2013)

McLaughlin T, Reaven G, Abbasi F, Lamendola C, Saad M, Waters D, Simon J, and Krauss RM. "Is there a simple way to identify insulin-resistant individuals at increased risk of cardiovascular disease?" Am J Cardiol 96: 399–404 (2005)

Mozaffarian D, Lemaitre RN, King IB, Song X, Huang H, Sacks FM, Rimm EB, Wang M, and Siscovick DS. "Plasma phospholipid long-chain ω-3 fatty acids and total and cause-specific mortality in older adults: a cohort study." Ann Intern Med. 158: 515–525 (2013)

Murguia-Romero M, Jimenez-Flores JR, Sigrist-Flores SC, Espinoza-Camacho MA, Jimenez-Morales M, Pina E, Mendez-Cruz AR, Villalobos-Molina R, and Reaven GM. "Plasma triglyceride/HDL-cholesterol ratio, insulin resistance, and cardiometabolic risk in young adults." J Lipid Res 54: 2795–2799 (2013)

Ramasamy R, Vannucci SJ, Yan SS, Herold K, Yan SF, and Schmidt AM. "Advanced glycation end products and RAGE: a common thread in aging, diabetes, neurodegeneration, and inflammation." Glycobiology 15: 16R–28R (2005)

Sears, B. *The OmegaRx Zone*. Regan Books. New York, NY (2002)

Tall AR. "C-reactive protein reassessed." N Engl J Med 350: 1450–1452 (2004)

APPENDIX G. POLYPHENOLS AND ORAC VALUES

Perez-Jimenez J, Neveu V, Vos F, and Scalbert A. "Identification of the 100 richest dietary sources of polyphenols." Eur J Clin Nutr 64: S112–S120 (2010)

Prior RL, Cao G, Prior RL, and Cao G. "Analysis of botanicals and dietary supplements for antioxidant capacity: a review." J AOAC Int 83: 950–956 (2000)

Index

Dutch Famine, 127–28
Dutch process cocoa, 84

E
Edmonton Obesity Scoring System, 155
eggs, xx, 19, 28, 118, 177
eicosanoids
  in cancer, 169
  in cellular inflammation, 131–32,
      139–40, 141, 142–43, 145
  clinical significance of, xiii, 6, 144–45
  gut health and, 119
  in hair growth, 174
  production of, 8–9, 11
eicosapentaenoic acid, 63, 68, 72
  in cellular inflammation, 148, 149
  health benefits of, 156
  in immune system, 146–47
  metabolic function of, 140–44
  see also AA/EPA ratio
endocannabinoids, 161
enzyme of life, 76, 101
EPIC study, 23
epigenetic change
  biological mechanism of, 126–27
  in current conceptualizations of diet,
      xvi
  definition of, xvi, 125–26
  in early childhood, 128
  in fetal development, 127–28
  industrialization of food supply and,
      130
  in intergenerational transmission of
      cellular inflammation risk,
      128–30, 133
  in intergenerational transmission of
      obesity risk, 161–62
  Zone diet to prevent negative effects of,
      130

F
fat, dietary
  calorie distribution in Zone diet, 20,
      21, 23, 28, 60
  cellular inflammation and, 140, 158
  historical evolution of human diet,
      33–35
  interesterified fats in, 112
  in Mediterranean diet, 32–33
  metabolic processing of, 115, 153–57

  in nuts, 73
  in processed foods, 108
  role of insulin in processing, 8, 13
  trans fatty acids in, 110–12
  in Zone Diet blueprint, xx–xxi, 17
fermented foods, 34
fetal development, epigenetic influences
    in, 127–28
fiber, dietary, 60
fibrosis, 150–51, 170
fish
  anti-inflammatory effects of
      consuming, 12
  as source of omega-3 fatty acids,
      62–64, 68, 142
  toxic contaminants in, 63–65
flax, 142
Food and Drug Administration, 110
frankincense, 82
free radicals
  beneficial, 93
  excess production of, 93
  fructose metabolization and, 115–16
  generation of, in metabolic process,
      94–95
  immune system production of, 93–94,
      147–48
  from omega-6 fatty acids, 10
  polyphenol role in controlling, 84–85,
      93, 94, 95, 98–99
fructose, 35, 114–16

G
galactose, 114, 116–17
garum, 34
gastric bypass surgery, 162–63
General Foods, 106
General Mills, 106
genetics
  in current conceptualizations of diet,
      xvi
  current scientific conceptualization of,
      126
  of plants, modification of, 85
  role of junk DNA in, 126, 127
  vulnerability to inflammation, 4
  see also epigenetic change
gene transcription factors, 98–99, 101,
      127, 146–47, 149, 155, 176–77
ghrelin, 160

glucose consumption, 114, 115, 116
glucose metabolism
of brain, 20, 114
in cancer metastasis, 170
carbohydrate consumption and, 155
cortisol secretion and, 158–59
insulin interactions in, 8, 18, 115, 116,
154, 158, 159–60
in sensation of hunger, 158–60
see also glycemic load
glutathione peroxides, 147–48
gluten and gluten sensitivity, 118,
119–21
glycemic load
from carbohydrates, 10–11
definition, 17–18
foods with, 17
goals of Mediterranean diet, 17–18,
20–21
insulin production and, 132
of meals, xx, 120
protein-to-glycemic load ratio, 22
of wheat, 120
glycerol, 154
glycosylated hemoglobin, 25, 182–83
grains
as cause of obesity, 119–20, 158
glucose content of, 73, 116, 199
health effects of, 18
as high-glycemic carbohydrate, 10–11,
17
historical evolution of human diet, 34
insulin production and, 8, 18
leaky gut syndrome and, 120–21
in Mediterranean diet, xx, 21, 33
negative health effects of, 10–11, 18,
83–84, 121
as polyphenol source, 73, 199, 201
in Zone Diet, xx
see also gluten
Grape-Nuts, 105–6
gut health
cellular inflammation and, 90–91
dietary strategy for, 91–92
hunger and, 160–61
industrialization of food supply and,
105
lactose intolerance and, 116–17
leaky gut syndrome, 91, 119–21, 146
obesity and, 89–90

role of bacteria in, 85–86, 88–89
role of polyphenols in, 86, 88, 89, 92,
188

H
hair health, 174–75
Harvard Medical School, 23, 102, 114,
159, 166
HbA$_1$c, 182
HDL cholesterol, 25, 168, 184
health
benefits of Mediterranean diet, 16, 28,
29–30
clinical markers of, 25–26, 179–85
effects of cellular inflammation, 9, 11,
13, 14–15, 19
effects of industrialization of food, 4
epigenetic transmission of risk factors
for, 127–30
metabolic processes of, 7–8
tax strategies to promote, 134–35
trends, 4–5, 15
of U.S. population, 25–26
see also gut health
health care system, 133–35
heart disease
cause of, 169
cellular inflammation and, 14
cholesterol and, 97
epigenetic causes of, 127–28
fibrosis in, 150–51
oxidation processes in, 19, 97, 168–69,
183–84
research in support of Mediterranean
diet, 29–30
saturated fats and, 112
trans fat consumption and, 111–12
Hershey, Milton, 106
high-fructose corn syrup, 35, 114–15
Hippocrates, vii, x, 134
histones, 126–27
hormonal system
in control of fat metabolism, 176
in control of hunger, 159–61
diet-induced inflammatory response
in, xiii, xv–xvi, 3–4, 145
effects of cellular inflammation in, 9,
165–66
evolution of, 144–45
goals of Zone Diet in, xix, 5–6

hormonal system (*cont.*)
    health effects of Mediterranean diet,
        17–18
    in maintenance of muscle mass, 175
    in normal metabolism, 7–8
    Zone state, xiv–xv
hunger
    alleviated by Zone diet, xxi, 17, 18, 20,
        163
    brain–gut communication and, 90
    determinants of sensation of, 8,
        157–63
hydroxyl, 93–94
hyperinsulinemia, 166, 167–68
hypochlorite, 93
hypoglycemia, 158
hypothalamus, 160, 167–68

I

immune system
    in cellular inflammation, 145–48
    free radial generation in, 93–94
    in gut health, 90–91
    inflammation-related disorders of,
        170
    innate functions of, 91, 145–46
industrialization of food supply
    epigenetic changes from, 130
    health outcomes of, 4–6, 10–11, 107,
        109
    in Mediterranean region, 34–35
    nutritional quality of food supply and,
        85, 106–7
    origins and development of, 82,
        105–7
    use of fats in, 108
    use of salt in, 108–9
    use of sugar in, 105–6, 107–8
    use of trans fats in, 110–11
inflammation
    biological processes in, 3, 9, 11,
        140–42
    genetic vulnerability to, 4
    goal of Zone Diet to control, xix, 5–6
    as hormonal response to diet, xiii,
        xv–xvi, 3–4, 9
    progression of, 165
    public health trends and, 4–5
    significance of, in medical health, 3,
        139

see also cellular inflammation;
        resolution of inflammation
insulin
    arachidonic acid formation and, 141
    carbohydrate consumption and, 115,
        116
    causes of increased levels of, 8, 10–11,
        73, 113, 132, 141
    clinical markers of healthy levels of,
        183–84
    controlling, to control cellular
        inflammation, 9
    dairy proteins and, 118
    in development of obesity, xv, 153–54,
        156–57
    in diabetes, 11, 168
    dietary control of, 155–56
    effects of food ingredients on secretion
        of, 188
    glycemic load of food and, 18, 20–21,
        115, 120
    health effects of, 8–9, 18–19, 91
    hunger and, 158, 159–60
    immune system response and, 91
    omega-6 fatty acids and, 8–9, 11,
        18–19, 107, 113
    resistance, 11, 13, 18, 91, 112, 113, 132,
        148, 157, 160, 166–71, 183–84
    weight gain and, 13
interesterified fats, 112
interleukin-6, 180
Italy, 69, 143

J

Japan, 68–69, 134–35, 143
Joslin Diabetes Center, 23, 166
Journal of Nutrition, 102

K

Keaton, Michael, xiv
Kellogg, John, 105, 106
Kellogg, Will, 106
Kellogg Company, 106
ketogenic diets, 156, 159, 167
ketones, 67, 71–72
kidney failure, 170
killer cells, 147
Kraft, James L., 106
Kraft Foods, 106
krill, 67

L

lactic acid, 117
lactose, 116–17
LDL cholesterol, 97–98, 168–69, 183–84
leaky gut syndrome, 91, 119–21, 146
legumes, 73, 194–95, 201
leptin, 160, 167–68
leucine, 177
leukotrienes, 119, 143, 149
life span, 72–73, 125
linoleic acid, 141–42
lipase, 166–67
lipodystrophy, 167
lipogenesis, 155, 157
lipotoxicity, 153
liver failure, 151, 168, 170
lobster, 63
LOX enzymes, 143, 145
Ludwig, David, xv–xvi
lunch, 35
   recipes, 38, 41, 44, 47, 50, 53, 56–57
Lyon Diet Heart Study, 29, 111

M

macrophages, 93, 94, 147, 168
macular degeneration, 71
maltose, 105–6
mammalian target of rapamycin, 176–77
Mapuche people, 76–77
maqui berry, 75–78, 202
Marco Polo, 34
margarine, 110–11
marijuana, 161
matrix metalloproteinases, 169, 174
Mayo Clinic, ix
McCay, Clive, 100–1
McCloy, Randall, 69–70
meals
   calorie distribution in Zone diet, 20, 28, 60
   carbohydrate content of ingredients for, 188–99
   historical evolution of, in Mediterranean region, 33–35
   oxygen radical absorption capacity of food ingredients, 188–202
   polyphenol content of food ingredients, 199–202
   recommended caloric load of, 161

schedule, 35
week-long menu plan, 60
Zone diet blueprint for, xix–xxi, 16–17
Mediterranean diet
   defining features of, ix–x, xvi–xvii, 6, 27–28
   health benefits of, 28–29
   historical evolution, 33–35
   research in support of, 28, 29–30
   weight control and, 29
   see also Mediterranean Zone Diet
Mediterranean Zone Diet
   for addressing manifestations of aging, 174, 175
   calorie distribution of meals in, 20–23, 28
   clinical markers of, 25–26, 179–85
   excessive weight loss with, 60
   expected results of, 24
   food pyramid, 32
   goals, 6, 23–24, 33, 35
   health benefits of, x, 16, 17–20, 62, 166
   paleo version, 60–61
   to prevent negative diet-induced epigenetic change, 130
   protein-to-glycemic load ratio of, 22
   research in support of, 23, 97, 102
   resources for users of, 137
   risk of excessive weight loss in, 21–22
   week-long menu plan, 60
   weight control and, x, 30–31, 163
memory, 70–71, 97–98
metabolic processes
   basic biology of, 7–8
   in development of obesity, 153–57
   diseases associated with disturbances of, 14
   effects of diet-induced inflammation, 9
   fetal programming of, 127–28
   generation of free radicals in, 94–95
metabolic syndrome, 166, 167–68
Mexico, 109
microRNA, 127
milk, 116–18
mono-unsaturated fat, xx–xxi, 28, 32–33
Montezuma, 82–83
Morandi, Daniela, 137
multiple sclerosis, 171

muscle mass, 175
myrrh, 82

N
National Weight Control Registry, 162
neo-glucogenesis, 158
neurological disorders
    causes of, 14
    fatty acid requirements of brain and, 144
    inflammation-related, 170–71
    omega-3 fatty acid deficiency and, 130
neuropeptide Y, 160
neutrophils, 93, 94, 147
New England Journal of Medicine, ix, 125
Nobel Prize in Medicine, xiii, 72, 90, 131–32, 139, 145
nuclear factor kappaB, 146–47, 148–49, 166, 169–70, 174, 180
nuts, xx–xxi, 73, 83, 102, 142, 201

O
oatmeal, 121
obesity
    caloric intake and, 157
    causes of, 69, 116, 119–20, 153–62
    cellular inflammation and, 11, 13–14
    definition of, 153
    epigenetic causes of, 127–28, 161–62
    epigenetic transmission of risk for, 129–30
    gut health and, 89–90
    high-fructose corn syrup consumption and, 114–15
    low-fat, high-carbohydrate diet and, xiii, xiv
    metabolically healthy, 154–55
    omega-6 fatty acid consumption and, 129–30
    trends, 4–5, 69, 129–30
    wheat consumption and, 119–20
olive oil, xx–xxi, 17, 29, 30, 74–75
omega-3 fatty acids
    anti-inflammatory role of, xvi, 12, 20, 69, 132, 142
    benefits of high-level supplements of, 69–73
    blood test for, 68–69
    to control hunger, 161
    conversion into eicosanoids, 145

effect on AA/EPA ratio, 181
fish as source of, 62–64, 68, 142
longevity and, 72–73
in management of inflammatory process, 94, 140, 141, 147, 149
in Mediterranean diet, 28
neurological outcomes of deficiency in, 130
oxidation, 67–68
recommended daily intake of, 63, 73
in resolution of inflammation, 9
supplements, 64–69, 71–72, 142
types of, 142. *see also specific type of*
omega-6 fatty acids
    blood test for, 68–69
    consumption trends, 10, 68
    controlling, to control cellular inflammation, xx–xxi, 9, 142
    conversion into eicosanoids, 145
    dietary sources of, 10
    health effects of, 8–9, 10, 18–19, 111–12, 132, 140, 141–42
    in industrialization of food supply, 106, 107, 141
    in infant formula, 128
    insulin and, 8–9, 11, 18–19, 107, 113, 132
    in intergenerational transmission of health risks, 129
    in Mediterranean diet, 28
    obesity and, 129–30
    in refined vegetable oil, 35, 141
    tax on production of, 135
OmegaRx Zone, The (Sears), xvi, 65, 69
oxidation and oxidation products
    in activation of cellular inflammation, 147
    of fatty acids in brain, 144
    in fish oil supplements, 67
    in insulin resistance, 168–69
    of LDL cholesterol, 97–98
    from omega-6 fatty acids, 10, 19
    polyphenols to prevent, 84–85
oxidative stress, 93
oxygen radical absorption capacity
    of food ingredients, 95–96, 188–202
    polyphenol levels and, 187, 199, 201
    recommended dietary goals, 98, 188
    significance of, 95, 187–88

wine, 199
in Cornaro's calorie-restricted diet, 100, 101
oxygen radical absorption capacity of, 196–97
polyphenols in, 34, 74, *74*, 75, 77, 83, 84, 91–92, 101, 199, 201
World Health Organization, 67

Y
yogurt, 34, 117

Z
Zone, The (Sears), xiii–xiv, xvi
Zone Diet
Atkins diet *versus*, 113–14
blueprint, xix–xxi, 16–17
goals of, xiv–xvi, xix, 5–6, 23–24
implications for health care system, 133–34
Mediterranean diet and, 30–31, 32–33
research in support of, xv–xvi, 23
see also Mediterranean Zone Diet

ABOUT THE AUTHOR

BARRY SEARS, PH.D., is recognized as one of the world's leading medical researchers on the hormonal effects of food. He is the #1 *New York Times* bestselling author of thirteen books, including *The Zone, Mastering the Zone,* and *Zone-Perfect Meals in Minutes.* His books have sold more than six million copies and have been translated into twenty-two languages. Dr. Sears has been a frequent guest on many national programs, including *20/20, Today, Good Morning America,* and *CBS Morning News.* A former research scientist at the Boston University School of Medicine and the Massachusetts Institute of Technology, he continues his research on the inflammatory process as the president of the nonprofit Inflammation Research Foundation in Marblehead, Massachusetts. The father of two grown daughters, he lives in Swampscott, Massachusetts, with his wife, Lynn.

zonediet.com

Facebook.com/TheZoneDiet

ABOUT THE TYPE

This book was set in Minion, a 1990 Adobe Originals typeface by Robert Slimbach. Minion is inspired by classical, old-style typefaces of the late Renaissance, a period of elegant and beautiful type designs. Created primarily for text setting, Minion combines the aesthetic and functional qualities that make text type highly readable with the versatility of digital technology.